To Julie

Happy horses gait better.

Anto Howe

Freedom to Gait

RELEASE YOUR HORSE INTO NATURAL EASY-GAIT

BY ANITA J HOWE

authorHOUSE®

AuthorHouse™
1663 Liberty Drive
Bloomington, IN 47403
www.authorhouse.com
Phone: 1-800-839-8640

First published by AuthorHouse   02/11/2011

ISBN: 978-1-4567-1618-9 (sc)
ISBN: 978-1-4567-1616-5 (e-b)

Library of Congress Control Number: 2010918958

Graphic Illustrations by Robert Knudsen

Printed in the United States of America
Bloomington, Indiana

This book is printed on acid-free paper.

Acknowledgements

Each of us has a pool of knowledge and understanding, built through life's experiences. As we are introduced to new ideas we analyze it to see if it *fits in* with our current pool of understanding. If so, we plug it in, adding to that pool much like we would a piece of jigsaw puzzle. If it doesn't quite fit we set it aside for later review before shucking it off into the pile of 'other suspicious thinking'. Sometimes in taking that second look we realize that if we turn it around this way, like the puzzle piece, it drops into place with our current understanding. Some ideas, however, still never quite make sense and get ejected as fad, rumor, or myth. As our understanding grows we begin to realize how little we knew in the beginning and to comprehend how great the ocean really is.

There are many people for me to thank for contributing to my journey and pool of knowledge regarding horses in general and gaited horses in particular who have made this work possible. While many of these people have influenced me directly, others have made contributions through their own literature, articles, books and educational media. These pieces add to the fundamental building blocks from which my own philosophies have evolved as well as often providing me with "holy cow!" moments of epiphany as I discover more truths about gaited horses. I hope to always be watching and listening for those fresh and innovative thoughts so my own journey may never end and my pool continues to grow.

I wish to recognize these people below as having made significant influences to my understanding and life with gaited horses.

Bruce Almeida: Working one on one with Bruce during his last years with us was a huge turning point in helping me understand how classical horsemanship is deserved by, and THE most successful tool for, the gaited horse. Bruce was constantly challenging me to be patient and persistent in my training and conditioning of the horse (and myself) while assuring me that the end result is well worth the effort; that any ignored holes in the horse's training will come back to bite you in the …(ahem) behind!

Tom Dorrance: Along with his brother Bill, I consider both of these gentlemen to be fathers of modern natural horsemanship. Tom's book ***True Unity*** will always be on my shelf. Before becoming clinicians, they were trainers; before trainers they were riders and students of the horse… but always they were horsemen!

Ray Hunt: Having learned from the best, Ray gave us a lucid and eloquent interpretation of the Dorrance training philosophies, while adding his own insights and experiences. His book ***Think Harmony with Horses*** will inspire anyone to a greater connection with their horse.

Lee Ziegler: Lee's book _**The Easy Gaited Horses**_ as well as her ever-patient explanations and thoughts on gaiting and biomechanics were an inspiration and an opened door for me.

Gary Lane: Gary is a superb sound trainer from Kentucky who has been a true gift to me in sharing his insight into the culture of the modern show world as well as being a constant and patient sounding board for training thoughts and methods. I highly recommend his book _**Training the Gaited Horse From the Trail to the Rai**_l. Thanks buddy, for always being willing to listen, discuss and jump in with both feet on behalf of the horse.

Liz Graves: Bless you Liz for your constant assurance that we can all be better to, and for, our horses; for your persistent and patient viewpoint that the horse should always come first, and your insistence that we should each earn our spurs as riders and equestrians; and finally thanks for your insights into all things Gait.

Dr. Deb Bennett: offers an authoritative guide to all sincere trainers (professional or not) into the complex subject of equine biomechanics, classical training as well as the history of all things horse. Her online articles and internet forums at Equine Studies Institute as well as her patient and succinct explanations _are_ a gift to those who wish to learn.

There are many other authors, researchers and trainers that I highly recommend and have benefited from. Please visit my website at www.naturalwalkinghorse.com for my personal list of recommended reading from which I believe you too can add to your pool of knowledge.

Introduction

The naturally gaited horse is not a myth and very attainable for almost anyone. An *overwhelming majority of* horses bred for gait can find a relaxed and smooth easy gait within their conformation. I would posit that even a significant majority of the partial (grade) bred gaited horses are likewise fully capable of finding a naturally free and balanced gait that has nothing to do with how they are shod.

Far too much of the currently available advice on gait is about how to mechanically alter a horse. For genuine happiness, comfort and true brilliance at gait your horse must learn to alter his own carriage becoming responsible for his balance and impulsion while you learn to release him into that gait, thereby providing him every opportunity to do so. When your horse is giving you the smooth ride you ask for, he should be carrying you with ease and comfort without pressure of any kind holding him into that gait. Training your horse through release allows him to be completely relaxed and happy while carrying you smoothly and willingly. He accepts responsibility for the gait he's carrying while secure in the understanding that the only pressure applied will be to ask him to change something. This security that you are keeping his wellbeing as a priority will go far in helping your horse to become a relaxed and thinking horse rather than a worried and reactive horse.

- **Part I** of ***Freedom to Gait*** delves into the biomechanics of equine movement *relating to gait* in great detail to offer you a *fundamental understanding* of how your horse carries himself and how best to unlock his gait potential.
- **Part II** gives you the ***tools*** you'll need to train through classical and natural horsemanship to engage his mind and help him become a willing partner that offers you his gait.
- **Part III** brings together the biomechanics and the horsemanship to provide you with a ***step by step plan*** to determine where your horse is having difficulty and how you can help him naturally correct his own carriage and balance, thereby correcting his gait. I discuss a variety of the most commonly seen gait problems as well as dedicate a healthy portion on developing the canter within your gaited horse.
- **Part IV** is dedicated to the naturally gaited walking horse, and helping those who wish to ***develop their horse's potential*** for the show ring *without gimmicks or mechanical enhancements.*

The easy gaits are as natural to your horse as the walk he was born with if *YOU* can learn to ***release him into gait***. I want you to understand and connect with his athletic potential for correct and balanced movement by understanding how he needs carry himself FREELY in self-carriage, taking responsibility for the gait he is giving you.

In passionately pursuing natural gait correction and training for many years, I can now offer solutions so you will never be forced to rely on inconsistent and questionable advice again. You can take direct responsibility for the relationship you have with your horse. ***It's time for horsemanship to return to the world of the gaited horse!*** With solid information, a little love and resolve, patience and persistence you too can free your horse to find his natural gait as you learn to become the partner he deserves.

Thanks for reading and happy gaiting!

Anita Howe

Contents

Part I – EASY GAITS DEFINED

By Anita J Howe

To analyze and understand gait we must breakdown how horses use individual parts of their bodies and how those individual parts relate to each other and work together. Lacking generally accepted standards within the gaited horse industry I have compiled what I term *Elements of Gait* to clarify and label definitive characteristics of equine movement as it relates to gait.

While some of these **elements** are more variable and influenced by the conformational structure of the horse, others are more definitive and pinpoint what a horse is doing, how he's balancing and which muscles are contracting and releasing. My goal is to help you understand each of these elements by breaking down each primary gait for easier comprehension of the biomechanics involved. That knowledge becomes a powerful tool in knowing what gait your horse is carrying at any given time allowing you to help him alter and improve that gait.

I cannot stress strongly enough that there is ABSOLUTELY NOTHING that happens with a horse's hooves that does not originate with his back, hips and shoulders. Also everything that happens to and with his hooves is directly influenced by his overall balance. Simply put **gait happens in the body and not the feet.** So no matter what you nail on his hooves, no matter how long you grow or angle those hooves, these changes will only marginally influence the end product but ***will never actually change his gait***. A person can nail on five pound tungsten steel shoes to a horse's front hooves to change the placement, break-over and delay the front stride enough to break-up a hard pace into a stepping pace, but what you need to realize is that THE HORSE IS STILL CARRYING THE PACE WITHIN HIS BODY. True alteration of gait comes from a horse's support structure, and is influenced only through his balance, his posture and conditioning. The voluntary correction of his posture, not the skills of the farrier changes his gait.

Trying to pinpoint the exact moment one gait alters to or becomes another is like trying to divide the colors of a rainbow. With a moderately trained eye many riders can tell when a horse is doing a nice rack as opposed to a good flatfoot walk. However, most will have difficulty in distinguishing a running walk that is slightly lateral in its timing from a stepping pace that has some headnod to it. IT'S IMPORTANT TO REMEMBER THAT THESE GAITS CAN, AND DO, MORPH INTO EACH OTHER VERY SEAMLESSLY. That is why we need better labels and definitive standards. These elements of gait give us tools to standardize what we're seeing and feeling. Definitive gait standards through these characteristics provide us with a better understanding of how a horse is using his body, as well as what is correct or incorrect for the different gaits. It also clarifies how we can help a horse correct his carriage to alter, improve or totally change his gait.

Chapter 1 – Five Elements of Gait

- Posture and Balance
- Head and Neck Attitude
- Weight Transfer / Hoof Support
- Timing (Lift and placement)
- Speed

POSTURE

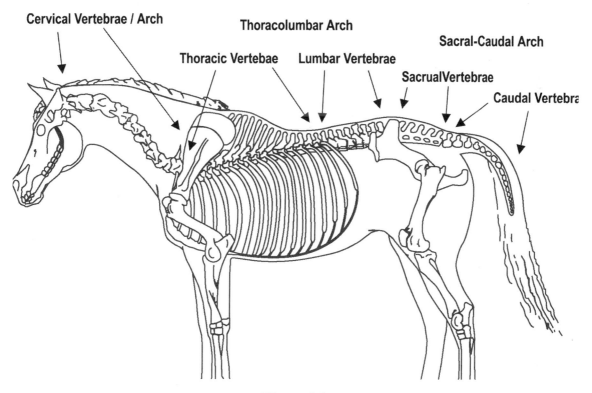

Cervical Vertebrae / Arch

Thoracolumbar Arch

Sacral-Caudal Arch

Thoracic Vertebae   Lumbar Vertebrae

SacrualVertebrae

Caudal Vertebra

Figure 1.1

The core of a horse from spine-to-abdomen, side-to-side and front-to-back, is able to move in a variety of directions with the vertebrae of the spine being uniquely constructed to allow a limited amount of flexibility while remaining strong for support. Though core movement is limited to only a few inches it has direct authority of not only his balance, but the use of his limbs so consequently the attitude of his core and its resulting balance are of critical influence over what gait a horse is carrying himself in. After all, the back supports everything else. Get a horse to change his posture and he *will* change his balance and gait. For the savvy eye the attitude carried through his core tells the tale of both cause and effect of gait.

There are three distinct arches of support within the spinal structure of equidae. The cervical arch of the neckline, the thoracolumbar arch from the withers to the L-S joint and finally the sacral/caudal arch of the loins all three play a role in balance, carriage and collection of a horse. Both the cervical and the sacral/caudal arches more directly affect

THE IMPORTANCE OF BALANCE

Balance is probably the most significant of all gait features when we're asking a horse to be deliberate and exact in the way he's carrying himself and the rider. I believe it to be the most distinctive characteristic to differentiate a quality gait from a mediocre or sub-standard gait. Front-to-back balance encompasses the engagement of the hindquarters vs. lightness of the fore and how he shares his weight between his supporting pairs of limbs. Balance directly affects the horse's ability to collect as well as his overall athleticism. Almost all quadrupeds balance between all four legs, but equidae are physically proportioned so that more than 60% of their standing body weight (and that of the rider) is supported with their forelegs leaving their hindquarters to be used as their engine for forward impulsion. I always relate it to a rear wheel drive car where all the forward push or drive comes from the rear wheels while the front wheels support the bulk of the engine and chassis weight.

The intrinsic carriage of a horse's spine allows them a limited amount of shift within their front to back balance and their muscle

balance front-to-back and athletic capacity, while the thoracolumbar arch is more directly responsible for the timing, lift and placement of his legs and therefore his footfall. Our ability to help our horse alter the way he uses these vertebral arches AND THEIR SUPPORTING MUSCULATURE is a key component in helping horses change, improve and even polish the brilliance of their gait and balance.

There are actually two distinct elements of the horse's carriage that are so interconnected and interdependent they often work as one though the savvy rider can learn to identify and isolate the individual affects and learn to train a horse to isolate and modify each as a distinct characteristic of gait. These elements are front-to-back balance and the posture of the core.

conditioning and training directly affects their ability to do so. Dr. Deb Bennett talks about three arches of support within the spine of a horse in her article titled *The Ring of Muscles Revisited* copy write 2008. I highly recommend this article that is available for view on her website equinestudies.org.

These supporting arches are capable of limited individual movement but are so interconnected through the musculature that they affect each other and often work in concert. The cervical arch and the thoracolumbar (T-L) arch often act in unison, so that when we ask a horse to release the dorsal muscles of his neck to lower his head, he will often release the dorsal muscles along his core T-L arch as well. Last, and most posterior, is the sacral-caudal arch from the sacrum through the tail dock. This arch is responsible for engaging to coil the loins or releasing to allow the hind legs to lag somewhat behind. It is my experience that the sacral-caudal arch operates with slightly more independence from the more forward two spinal arches, particularly in gaited horses.

The action of each of these structures upon

the horse is very distinct and your recognition of these movements will be a tremendous advantage in working with your horse.

In the gaited breeds it is not uncommon to observe a coiling of the loins while the lower neck and core are being carried more hollowed. I see this most often with performance walking horses and feel this accounts for their ability to keep the hind quarters engaged in a walking stride while the timing is carried lateral and the shoulders are not lifted.

When lifting or rounding the cervical arch near the base of his neck (which some refer to as lifting the lower neck or lifting the withers) a horse stretches his poll forward. This movement doesn't just lift the withers and lightens his fore; it encourages a release of the dorsal muscles of his core as well as a coiling of his loins that are both essential to a sweeping walking stride. This singular lifting movement, so very desirable in almost every equine sport, enables a horse to reach under for stronger backend impulsion while producing a measurable shift in balance toward his hindquarters.

Conversely when the poll rises higher, the muscles along the top of the neckline contract and shorten to counteract any forward stretch and tends to hollow the base of the neck in front of the withers. This lowering of the withers not only promotes a heavy-on-the-fore balance, but may cause the dorsal muscles of the core to contract and hollow as well. Both actions actually encourage the loins to uncoil to produce strung-out hindquarters, tension through the hips and disengagement of the walking swing or stride. When all three spinal arches drop into hollow posture a horse will invariably load his weight to the fore even more so than when standing square at ease. Visualize the rocker of a rocking chair. This rocker shape is how a hollow horse is balancing his weight, and like a rocker he will tend to focus that weight (ground support) toward a centralized point that, lacking any outside influence, will be his forehand. When a horse stands with his dorsal muscles relaxed and stretched he will quite naturally balance more toward the distal quadrants of his legs. The higher he raises his head and contracts the dorsal muscles for that lift, the more his natural counter-balance will be to nose out on the front and lighten behind with an uncoiled sacrum, all of which further concentrates his weight onto his forelegs.

A rider mistakenly attempting to force a horse to lighten on his fore by increasing bit pressure and framing his head through the bit creates a **Catch 22** effect that actually contributes to his imbalance rather than helps it. Eventually this continued bit pull or framing will result in the horse leaning into severe pressure where the rider seems to be holding up the front of the horse. Note: a rider can never actually lift a horse while riding on that horse's back because physics tells us that any pressure applied through the reins will be redirected to equal and opposite pressure downward through the rider's seat and stirrups. This severe and totally mistaken effort actually causes a disconnect through the horse's midline, as well as awkward and seriously stiff carriage. We will address this in greater detail in the training chapters.

When hollowness occurs, weight shifts to the fore creating an anchoring affect which becomes a tremendous disadvantage for lateral movement, bending or rapid directional changes and will greatly inhibit a horse's athleticism. For this reason the lifting of the lower neck or withers is much sought for in almost all equestrian disciplines. You simply cannot have real collection and brilliant athleticism without it. This essential lightness not only provides fluid balance but encourages quality backend engagement for greater impulsion.

COLLECTION

Collection is a gathering from back to front through a horse's body in preparation for balanced impulsion. I love the analogy of a young child's first time in a batter's box playing T-ball. He stands there flatfooted, straight legged and swings at the ball with very little power and less accuracy. Later, after a few years of Little League practice he stands with his feet further apart, balanced forward on the balls of his feet, his knees bent, leaning forward at the waist, his arms held high and his head tilted in. He's learned to collect himself to add both power and accuracy by swinging not just with his arms but with and through his entire body. He has collection.

Much like this youngster, our horse can learn to gather his energy and power for deliberate athletic movement. Collection can be light with a simple coiling of his loins, or it can be moderate by adding a lift of the lower neckline to lighten his fore. It can also be extensive by finally adding a rounding up of his core.

Please note that at **NO TIME** do I relate collection to a positioning of the horse's face because *headset has nothing to do with collection*. Many people make the mistake of thinking headset is collection, but the reality is that overly setting a horse's face on or behind the vertical can actually inhibit real collection by locking the lower neckline into the down and hollow posture. When a rider forces or frames a horse's head high, and restricts their face onto vertical alignment from this elevated position the cervical vertebrae cannot telescope forward and outward to release the lower neck and allow it to lift or lighten at the withers. The horse is forced to carry himself heavy on his fore because the rider has taken away his sole method of lifting it from within his own self carriage.

CORE POSTURE RELATIVE TO GAIT

Simply put, the attitude and posture through a horse's thoracolumbar vertebral arch *has the most direct influence over the timing of both lift and placement of his individual or paired footfalls.* This core area is found behind the shoulders or withers and in front of the sacrum or loins. Some maintain its alignment and carriage to be the most key element of gait. I personally acknowledge its importance, however I feel that balance as well as engagement of the supporting pairs to be just as vital to the gait being produced as well as the quality of that gait.

Some trainers and clinicians assert that the VERTEBRAL ALIGNMENT is directly responsible for the timing or pairing of the legs during a horse's stride rotations. I have found rather that it's the engagement and use of the CORE MUSCLE GROUPINGS instead of the vertebral alignment to be most responsible for the pairing or isochronal usage of the individual limbs. The difference is subtle but important when it comes to training. There are many gaited breeds that will carry a naturally hollow alignment of their vertebrae due to their conformation, even while relaxed and grazing along *in the isochronal timing of most relaxed walks*. It is also common to see non-gaited horses easily trotting while hollow. Both these instances seem to support that it is not the actual level, rounded or hollow ALIGNMENT, but rather a dominant engagement of dorsal or ventral muscling or even the relaxed and alternating isochronal usage of both that contributes to variances of timing.

The facts are that as a horse executes a rounding up of his core he will tend to utilize a dominance of ventral (abdominal) muscling to do so. His ventral muscles contract, shorten and tighten greater than the dorsal muscles.

Often the dorsal muscles will relax and stretch out as this happens, but sometimes they will maintain a limited contraction in opposition which creates greater tension throughout the core. In either case the key element is that THE VENTRAL MUSCLES WILL DOMINATE in what I refer to as **ventral dominance**. This greater shortening of the belly line muscles will often produce a rounding up through the topline. Conversely, when a horse drops his topline more hollow he will use a dominance of dorsal muscles (dorsal dominance). While in a neutral carriage both dorsal and ventral muscles are clearly firing in alternating, non-dominant fashion.

In illustration consider the central arch of a horse much like an archer's bow where the MUSCLE GROUPINGS act like a string to alter the alignment of the vertebrae (the stem of the bow). The nature of all muscles is to shorten when they contract, and lengthen as they relax. When muscles shorten above the spine, as in dorsal dominance, they shorten and pull together. As they shorten the topline drops into hollow, or more hollow alignment similar to how we would arch our back. Conversely, when the ventral muscles below and along the belly contract and shorten, it not only encourages the dorsal muscles to release but this ventral dominance tends to round or lift upward the spinal alignment through the core. When neither muscle group overwhelms the core and engage in an alternating sequence of contractions and releases, a more neutral and released topline is observed. This released topline produces more fluid and relaxed movement in the gait being carried.

In the following sections I will discuss how each of these core attitudes affects the timing and usage of the leg pairings. To learn more details about the physiology, skeletal and musculature usage I recommend visiting Dr. Deb Bennett's **Equine Studies Institute** online for informative articles on these equine systems.

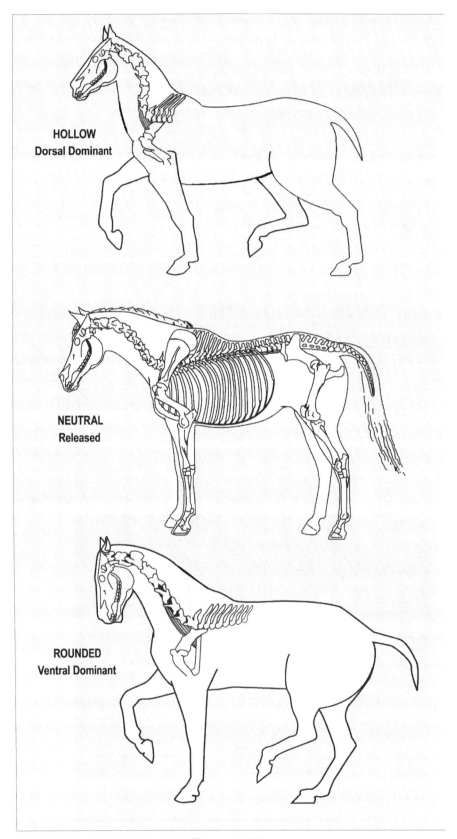

Figure 1.2 1

DORSAL DOMINANCE

Some of you may already be aware that when a horse is moving in more lateral gait (pace, step-pace and many racks) that his tendency will be to carry his core in a more hollow posture. Commonly referred to as ventroflexion, literally meaning ***toward the ventrum or belly***; this is a core posture where the spine and abdomen have dropped, much as we would arch our back pushing our abdomen forward.

The hollow back is often carried with tremendous tension and brace throughout the spine if the back of the horse is under stress. When that core hollows the abdomen to stretches downward sometimes even causing the loin to disengage (uncoil) and allowing the hind legs to string out behind. It is quite common for the head and upper neck to lift high in front as those dorsal muscles shorten and contract.

Bracing occurs anytime muscles are contracting in opposition to each other (antagonism) and actually serves to strengthen the topline. Bracing through his core makes it more very difficult for a horse to keep his hips and shoulders loose and rolling. Properly alternating contractions and releases of both ventral and dorsal muscles is needed for the evenly timed four-beat gaits to occur.

The hollow core carriage predisposes many gaited horse to hard pace. I believe there are a couple of reasons for this. The primary factor being the dominance of dorsal muscles engaged in support of that hollow posture. These muscles are aligned mostly lengthwise along either side of the spine much of which is above the transverse (wing-like) processes of the vertebrae. Whereas the ventral muscling has a great deal more diagonal alignment beneath the belly or core one would assume to provide greater support for vital organs. A dominance of these lengthwise aligned dorsal muscles creates greater support for the legs to

pair up laterally, while a dominance of the more diagonally aligned ventral muscles encourages and allows a more diagonal pairing. This is just a broad overview of a very complex system of support.

The second reason this posture supports lateral pairing relates more to the skeletal structure itself. The vertebrae of the spine are shaped with upward angled processes that as the dorsal muscles dominate shorten and pull together. These processes when contracted together limit flexibility by producing rigidity through the topline. This rigidity, while vital and necessary for protection of the horse's core, decreases his ability for side to side bend. It is important to note that some side-to-side bend through the core is essential for both isochronal and diagonal gaits by allowing the legs on each side of the body to approach and retreat from each other during the stride rotation. This side-to-side movement is needed for every intermediate gait *EXCEPT* the pace. It is only when pacing that both legs on each side of the equine body swing with synchronicity or complete lateral pairing. At the complete diagonal pairing of the trot the same legs on each side move in total opposition to each other. This opposite movement requires the muscles along their sides to allow the legs to come together and to separate during each stride rotation. Simply put there is a side-to-side movement needed for both diagonal and isochronal gaits which is made much more difficult with a rigidly hollow topline.

Hollow posture further interferes with a horse's ability to collect. Collection is a gathering through a horse's body from back to front in preparation for balanced impulsion. The hollow topline is the antithesis of a collected topline and as such it inhibits fluid balance and athletic motion for anything other than a straight forward bolt. That is also why a hollow horse tends to be stiff and less able to manage lateral bending through their core. The front-to-back stiffness is resistant to lateral bend and promotes a forward balance. That is why the hollow horse often tends to fall over his shoulder when asked for turns rather than allowing his barrel to bend and the shoulder to properly lift up for stepping in with lightness and balance. This is evident when a hollow horse is asked for a side step or leg yield and he drops onto his inside shoulder giving the rider a sensation of falling into the turn.

While equine foreleg conformation can allow a horse to roll or angle both legs together at the shoulder toward the side for quick changes of direction at high speed, a slower and more deliberate shift in balance allows and encourages him to achieve lightness on the fore, using the haunches to support himself in a brilliant execution of lateral movement. This kind of haunch engagement and front end lightness may best be witnessed in cutting horses as they quickly alter their direction while working cows or by reining horses executing haunch spins as well as a multitude of other equestrian maneuvers.

There are a vast number of influences which can and do contribute to horses carrying themselves hollow. Starting horses under saddle far too young is certainly high on that list. Immature backs are often forced to brace when ridden before they are strong enough to support the rider's weight. Hollowness may also occur from pulling on the bit to frame the head into headset and riding with too much constant bit pressure. Positioning the saddle too far back places weight on the unsupported lumbar vertebrae causing the spine to drop and dorsal muscles contract in support. Rider positioning may be another culprit so watch that chair seat folks because shifting our weight further back in the saddle creates much the same effect. It's sometimes in the very nature of some horses to assume this hollow posture during their more fright and flight worry modes. Throwing their heads high and noses out to increase their distance vision produces this hollow, rigid and straight posture. Then of course we are sometimes dealing with a horse's natural conformational tendencies. Whatever the cause, we need to be aware of it so we might take steps to avoid it and learn how to correct.

VENTRAL DOMINANCE

When we watch well trained dressage horses move in a collected trot, we most often see a rounder dorsi-flexed core. This core posture is what is most desired and trained for in that discipline and is most closely associated with *TRUE COLLECTION*, better enabling the horse for upward and lofting motion. When we note a rounded topline in a gaited horse we will most often be observing one that, indeed, shows that same tendency to move in very diagonal timing (toward the trot) such as a foxtrot, or fox-rack (a rack with a diagonal or broken trot timing), and sometimes even in an actual hard trot.

The rounded topline is not as braced nor quite as rigid as the hollow topline because the vertebrae are more released as the horse relaxes his dorsal muscling while engaging more contraction (or shortening) of the ventral muscling. Keep in mind that a horse carries an average of 57% of his weight through the core area of his body between the withers and the sacrum. When the topline muscles release strong ligaments along the spine stretch taut in support allowing the vertebrae themselves to telescope slightly apart. This action transforms the spine of the horse from a braced and rigidly hollow frame to a released, stretched and somewhat more flexible suspended support.

Because real collection comes not only from releasing the dorsal muscles but also from engaging the ventral muscles to produce a posture with some essential tension through the core. Collection means a spring coiled and prepared for action. The rounded posture allows the horse to gather himself; to collect for forward impulsion and athletic endeavors. It is a posture that permits the horse to balance himself better because his legs can be gathered beneath with quality engagement on all four corners. You will hear me repeatedly say that diagonal timing and rounded posture is more supportive for more upward loft while remaining more stable at the slower speeds and the lateral postures are more conducive for fast forward and straighter movement. Roundness allows the horse to lift better out of the shoulders while his released topline

LEVEL / RELEASED

The level or neutral core is where those gaits with more isochronal timing will occur. The level spine allows for a more relaxed carriage, and generally means much less bracing. Less tension or bracing allows for easier independent use of each quadrant of the horse. Watch a horse grazing in the pasture and you'll see a neutral top line; one that's completely relaxed (not braced, not dorsi-flexed and not ventroflexed) and that horse will invariably be walking along with a four-beat lift and placement regardless of his conformation. The level and released topline is the natural posture of the walk for *any horse of any breed*. Solid back conformation allows the muscles of the spine and abdomen to be conditioned to easily support a rider with less brace required. A strong back enables the horse to maintain this neutral posture for easier four-beat gait without the muscles pulling the gait away from isochronal evenness. It is vital to understand that the stronger and more conditioned the dorsal and ventral muscles become *AT THE WALK*, the easier

allows him to achieve improved lateral bend. The essential tension involved with a very rounded and collected core tends to impede relaxed movement that allow all four corners to work independently by increasing tensions emanating from the underline (ventral) just as the hollow core will likewise impede independent and even timing because of tension produced in the topline (dorsal).

Please note that while rounding of the mid-back arch is part of real collection, it is **not the only** characteristic of a much desired movement that involves *ALL THREE* arches of spinal support. For more detailed discussion please refer to the chapter on **Collection or Headset**.

it will be for that horse to carry that neutral posture and even timing to greater speeds for intermediate gaits as well. This is precisely why I advocate the walking gaits as the foundation training and conditioning gait for any horse of any discipline. Successful movement and responsiveness at the walk will lay the foundation for more successful intermediate and speed gaits.

It is worth note that a further benefit of the released posture, neutral topline and independent movement of the walking gait is to highlight any stresses or lamenesses that a horse may be experiencing. Once your eye is trained and the feel of your seat is educated, the released movement of the walk will allow us to recognize uneven movement. Any uneven motion will enable us to better recognize that there is a problem but also to isolate and identify which quadrant it relates to. I speak of the seat and feel because *feel can be much more sensitive than the human eye* in identifying imbalances and non-symmetrical movement.

HEAD AND NECK ATTITUDE

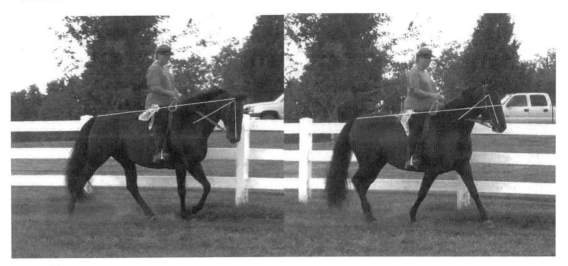

Figure 1.3 Papa's Midnight Pearl

The position and use of the head and neck are a vital part of a horse's posture, as well as a critical tool for the savvy trainer. Because the head and neck carriage is *a reflection of the rest of his body* it is, in my opinion, the easiest indicator of exactly how a horse is balancing and carrying himself. While I will continue to stress that head and neck attitude is a product of core posture and balance, many people do not realize how huge an *influence* it is to ask a horse to change his carriage, nor how to utilize it as a training tool beyond frame or force.

A horse uses his head and neck weight to not only balance, but to counterbalance and add thrust to his body's natural movement in whatever direction he needs to move. Have you ever tried to jog uphill without pumping your arms? Jogging is always more difficult when you restrict the natural counterbalancing motion of your arms, but even more so when you are putting tremendous thrust into your legs as when going uphill. We naturally help our push and thrust by offsetting it with the swing of our arms and thereby reduce the strain on our leg muscles.

Biomechanics of a horse's structure allows him to use what is essentially his most mobile and significantly weighted appendage to offset the shifting and thrust of his legs. Whether it's needed to add power to his forward stride, to throw upward for rearing in battle or to lower his center of gravity to add push to his front legs for a sideways dive to head off an escaping calf, the head and neck are the single biggest tool for the horse to quickly rebalance, change direction or add power to the rest of his body.

The head and neck of the gaited horse, therefore, not only helps us define what gait he is currently engaged in by being a product of that gait, but becomes an important means to encourage a change in his balance and carriage. By understanding how a horse should carry himself in various gaits, we can extrapolate how he needs to utilize this critical balancing tool to alter that gait.

We can also learn to read his head and neck attitude to better define how he may be balancing incorrectly. How he carries and uses this significant area in front of his shoulders can tell us how he's counterbalancing, whether he's stiff and braced, heavy on the fore, light on the fore, etc. Though head and neck usage does not produce gait, *IT IS A PRODUCT OF BOTH GAIT AND BALANCE* that can tell us exactly how a horse is carrying himself.

Head and neck usage is also the first place I carefully watch to help detect unbalanced movement produced by lamenesses. If the headnod is not evenly deep on both sides of his stride I can begin to isolate where the horse is experiencing discomfort. The rule of thumb is ***down on sound*** so a horse will dip his head lower as the sound leg or legs are weight bearing and more shallow as those legs experiencing pain are bearing his weight or engaging for thrust. Because the headnod is driven by the hind legs a similar alteration of the headnod occurs for those limbs much as

it does for the forelegs.

Isolating which area of the body is sore or lame is the first step to resolving the issue. Don't be embarrassed if you have difficulty with this determination early on. Even experienced veterinarians need to carefully watch to isolate a sore limb. Just knowing there is a problem is a great start and should you see evidence of a stride that is asymmetrical or a headnod that is uneven, I advise you to have your veterinarian follow up with a complete lameness exam as early as possible.

Weight Transfer and Hoof Support

Weight transfer

Gait does not happen in the legs of a horse. Knowledgeable horse owners understand that there are no muscles below the knees and hocks of a horse's legs, only bone, tendon and ligament covered by skin. All of the muscles responsible for moving their legs are situated in the upper legs, the shoulders, hips and through their core. Simply put *that* is where gait happens, not below his knees and hocks. One common theme you will hear me repeat throughout this book or my clinics, is that gait has nothing to do with what's nailed on the hooves of the horse. While you *may* be able to slightly break up a pacing horse's timing by mechanically altering his hooves, you will not change the fact that in his body he is still executing a pace. It is only through changing the use of the muscles above that you can get the horse to change the gait he is performing. So when we're discussing the mechanics of weight transfer and hoof support phases we must look to his hips, shoulders and back for *that* is where his leg motion originates.

Weight transfer is the characteristic of how a horse transfers or shifts weight from one leg of a SUPPORTING PAIR to the other. A horse has two pair of supporting legs. For this discussion please realize that a pair of limbs

that alternate support for one portion of their body (such as the hips or the shoulders) is a supporting pair that can be compared relative to our one pair of supporting legs.

Our supporting pair of legs may transfer weight via stride, step, hop, skip or jog. Similarly a horse transfers weight between the hooves of his supporting pair of legs with a walking (both-hooves-on-the-ground) step, or an aerial (no-hooves-on-the-ground) leap or jog. For my explanation we'll call it suspended or non-suspended weight transfer.

By studying what happens with our own hips and pelvis (our primary weight support joint) and the changes occurring there as we alter from a walking gait to a jogging gait. Let's examine…

As we walk our lower back and hip muscles loosen and release so that we are able to roll our hips. This rolling action is what allows us to do a number of things:

- To lift our non-supporting leg with less bend for ground clearance and forward movement. We distribute the lift for ground-clearance between hip, knee and ankle for a more energy efficient, less exaggerated motion at this relaxed walking gait.

- To maintain an evenly balanced upper torso and avoid having to lift or suspend the majority of our weight as we stride.
- It allows us to place the striding foot on the ground before the weight bearing foot lifts off and to transfer our weight in a smooth rolling movement that is easier on our frame as well as more relaxed and energy efficient.

As we alter to a jogging step our lower back and hips need to brace so that our pushing leg has a firm support to loft our weight upward for that jog. The knee and ankle joints must engage first with more flex and then push as our weight is literally vaulted from foot to foot and *WE BECOME COMPLETELY AIRBORNE FOR A MOMENT, HOWEVER BRIEF.* This is referred to as an aerial phase, just as the time when our foot is in contact with the ground is a support phase. We expend significantly more energy in order to suspend our body mass upward for an aerial phase. The resulting movement is therefore more energy 'expensive' but enables us to greatly increase our forward speed. The walking gait is more energy conserving, and takes significantly less effort in pushing our weight forward by rolling our support from foot to foot.

Now take these human examples and apply them directly to how a horse uses his hips and shoulders that are his *SUPPORTING PAIRS.* In his walking gait he needs to loosen his hips and shoulders in a released rolling stride that allows him to *place both hooves of a supporting pair on the ground at the same time for a smooth shift of weight transfer, with NO aerial phase.* When he suspends his weight (jogs), his hips or shoulders need to brace for supporting the upward thrust of the lofting weight transfer in a suspended stride. This results in that brief moment of aerial phase as well as the shortened reach.

A horse's supporting pairs have the ability

to work independently of each other. Therefore the horse may suspend or not with *EITHER* his shoulders or hips; and this suspension, or lack of, directly affects as well as defines what gait they carrying. Sometimes it becomes very difficult to tell from the ground whether a horse is actually bracing and engaging his hocks or knees for upward loft because the action is so minute that at speed it is almost undetectable to all but the rider's feel or a video camera's stop-frame photography. One huge clue is that when a horse does brace their shoulders or hips a trained eye can often detect the shortened stride coupled with increased knee or hock action. But the real proof is in the feel. A sensitive rider can learn to feel even the smallest amount of float sensation as the horse begins to suspend during weight transfer, as well as a lessening of the hip and shoulder roll and reach. Each of these has a very unique feel from the saddle. Watching from the ground I instruct observers to study the head and neck in the front, as well as the tail dock in the rear. If the shoulders have braced the headnod will decrease or even cease, and if the hips have braced the tail dock will begin to show vertical jig rather than the side-to-side swing of the non-suspended walking stride.

A horse must brace his shoulders and hips to suspend during weight transfer with front *AND* back when trotting, pacing and racking. Which is why these are all considered gaits of full suspension. Note that full suspension gaits will generally be more energy expensive for your horse to carry long term.

During increases of speed in gait there is a natural characteristic of progression in both humans and quadrupeds. We can walk slowly or we can walk faster. We can jog slowly or we can sprint faster. In the progression of increasing speed and energy cost we would normally start with a slower walk and a shorter stride then gradually increase in speed by extending the stride as well as increasing the tempo *WHILE STILL MAINTAINING THE WALKING*

STRIDE. From there we progress into maximum walking speed, tempo and extension just before we transition to a jog. The characteristic I wish to highlight here is the tendency to go from maximum stride reach and extension to a *lesser reach* as we transition to the jogging step. Because the jog introduces an aerial phase as well as impact as we land our natural inclination is to first shorten our reach in order to reduce the stress to our joints as the loft, effort and impact are all added. Remember we're talking about a progression of energy and speed here. Of course we CAN immediately go to maximum sprint, but that is rarely the norm for people or our horses. Maximum acceleration usually only happens to a horse when he is startled and reacting in fear in order to escape from danger. From horseback the expected progression of speed and energy is for a horse to first shorten his forward reach as he transitions into the jog, or suspended weight transfer. This characteristic becomes particularly important to those who seek to train their horse's walking gaits for the show ring and maximize their stride potential.

Hoof Support

Hoof support refers to whichever hooves are actually in contact with the ground, supporting weight at any given moment during the stride cycle of the horse. Represented numerically, it is expressed in a sequence to indicate how the horse's (and rider's) weight is being supported throughout a single stride cycle. Some gait enthusiasts will consider it an element of gait in and of itself. However, I am of the belief that hoof support is a product of timing and weight transfer rather than a definitive element by itself: timing + weight transfer = hoof support.

When a horse is moving in a walking gait, without any suspended weight transfer, you should see both hooves of a supporting pair on the ground at their moment of weight transfer; *a supporting pair being either the front pair or the hind pair of hooves*. During an isochronal walking gait as weight is being transfer on one supporting pair, the other pair should be exactly mid-stride and have only one of those hooves in contact with the ground creating the signature three hoof support of the walk.

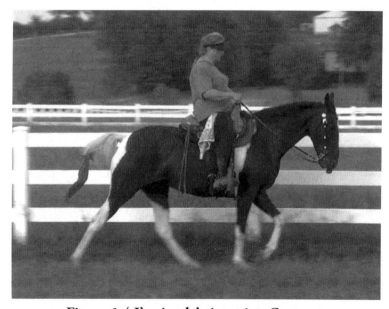

Figure 1.4 I'm Angle's Amazing Grace

When a horse is moving you will see both hooves of a supporting pair on the ground at the same time *ONLY* during a non-suspended transfer of weight where the supporting joint (shoulders or hips) is loose and rolling.

The two beat pace, the four beat rack and the two beat hard trot all involve suspended weight transfer on both front and back supporting pairs; the foxtrot involves suspension in the rear only with non-suspension in the fore; and in a true walking gait there should be no suspension, front or back, only the rolling, energy efficient weight transfer with both hooves in contact with the ground.

The method of weight transfer **strongly defines** a horse's gait and is directly responsible for hoof support sequence for it takes the 1,2,3,4 of hoof placement coupled with the timing factor to produce the additional dimension of how many hooves are supporting at any given moment during the stride rotation.

Because it illustrates the method of weight transfer hoof supp0ort is also a definitive though often difficult to quantify element of gait. For example the isochronal walk of *any* horse will have a 3 hoof – 2 hoof – 3 hoof – 2 hoof support *SEQUENCE* as he moves through one full stride rotation; three hooves supporting, then 2 hooves, then 3, then 2 again. In a true walking gait there is never fewer than 2 hooves making ground contact. For convenience this hoof support is frequently expressed as 3-2-3-2, and illustrates the horse is transferring weight in a rolling, both-hooves-on-the-ground motion both front and behind. If any four beat gait includes a suspended weight transfer on either the front or the back (and many do) this will create a moment of single hoof support and will be reflected in the resulting

TIMING

Timing is probably the most easily recognized element of gait, the placement of which can be identified by most gaited horse

sequence. A foxtrot has suspended weight transfer on the back only and this produces a 3-2-1-2-3-2-1-2 sequence. Hoof support gives us another definition for each gait with both the pace and the trot producing a 2 – 0 – 2 – 0 sequence at the extreme poles of the gait scale. A trot is executed with absolute diagonal pairing of both lift and placement, while the pace has absolute lateral (same side) pairing. Any intermediate gait not having absolute pairing becomes four beat. We delve into this in greater detail in the following section on Timing.

The rack becomes a little trickier to define because it encompasses such a large range of variance from the shorter strided, shuffling step of the saddle-rack, to the faster single-foot and super reaching speed rack. The one thing that each of them will have in common is that at some point they will have a moment of *SINGLE HOOF SUPPORT FOR EACH OF THE FOUR HOOVES* during the stride cycle. The saddle racks will often resemble a shuffling intermediate walk, while the speed racks will be a truer single-foot gait. Both will exhibit a 2 – 1 – 2 – 1 sequence and should *NEVER HAVE THREE HOOVES ON THE GROUND TOGETHER*. The wide range of difference is a product of extension and speed in this same basic gait. While I think you could almost write a book about all the variables of the racking gaits alone, they all have these common characteristics:

- Fixed head carriage
- Rigid topline
- Suspended weight transfer fore and hind
- A moment of single hoof support for each hoof during the stride cycle
- Four beat placement of the hooves

enthusiasts with a little practice. Timing refers to the pattern or synchronization for both *LIFT AND PLACEMENT* of the hooves within each stride rotation; a stride rotation being one complete cycle of all four hooves making contact with the ground. Timing is how each leg relates to the other three as a horse walks or 'jogs' with his legs. The synchronization or pairing of the leg movements becomes a highly visible element that can help us define what gait is being performed. For consistency in discussion stride cycle illustrations are usually characterized as always starting with the left hind leg. *EVERY FOUR-BEAT EASY GAIT WILL HAVE A LEFT HIND, LEFT FRONT, RIGHT HIND, RIGHT FRONT HOOF SEQUENCE.*

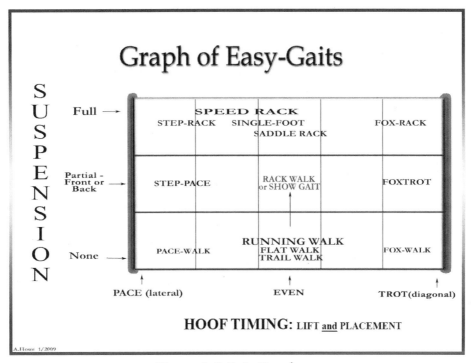

Figure 1.5 Gait Graph

While trot and pace are both two beat gaits, they are polar opposites on the 'timing scale' representing the extremes in either direction, with all four-beat easy gaits falling somewhere in between. The trot is executed with complete *diagonal pairing* a hind leg lifts and plants in synchronization with its diagonally opposite fore leg. The pace is executed with complete *lateral pairing* where a hind leg lifts and plants in synchronization with the same side fore leg. Both of these gaits exhibit a hind leg lifting and planting in total synchronization with a fore creating only two beats to be seen, heard and felt during each four hoof stride rotation. With the trot being diagonal and the pace lateral they represent the two beat extremes of timing. I frequently use the terms hard trot and hard pace as the true two-beat synchronization produces a very noticeable impact moment for the rider which confirms this two beat pairing. Those four-beat gaits directly in the middle of these extremes are referred to as isochronally timed, or evenly spaced in tempo 1 – 2 – 3 – 4 where each hoof lifts and plants individually and independently of each other in a rhythmic, evenly space beat. Isochronal gaits include all of the walking gaits (trail walk, flatfoot walk and the running walk). Many of the racking gaits (saddle rack, slow rack, single-foot and speed rack) *MAY* also be executed with isochronal timing. All of these are referred to as easy gaits because any breaking away from the pure two beat impact softens the ride. Even small offsets from the true two beat will create an easier impact and many non-gaited breeds can even be taught to soften their trots this way.

Pairing occurs when hoof beat intervals move away from evenly spaced or timed placement. It is when increased time elapses between some hoofbeats and others indicating that in one direction or another the hoofbeats are getting closer than others as evidenced by the shorter time intervals. When a horse moves with more diagonal pairing, such as with a foxtrot or foxrack, the diagonal hooves (opposite side fore and hind) pair up to lift and place *MORE CLOSELY TO EACH OTHER WITH LESS TIME BETWEEN THOSE BEATS*. Diagonal pairing should not be confused with the absolute synchronization as seen with the hard trot.

Similarly, a stepping pace and many racking gaits are closer to the pace, and show lateral (same side fore and hind) pairs being lifted and planted closer together, giving the horse lateral pairing in a four-beat gait. Both of these are examples of gaits that move away from evenly spaced tempo or beat, and closer to the two-beat polar extremes.

Timing can be determined from still photography or graphic representations as well. We can read timing in any gait image by studying the placement of the legs by their relationship to each other at any particular moment. It is by far easiest when one supporting pair or the other is at the weight transfer, both-hooves-on-the-ground moment.

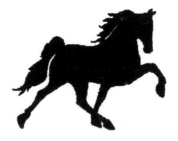

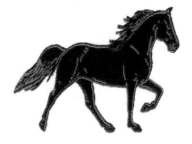

Figure 1.6 TWH Icons

Now compare the graphic of two commonly seen Walking Horse icons shown in figure 1.6. One is the performance horse icon (top), the other a pleasure horse icon (bottom). *THESE IMAGES ARE BOTH INTENDED TO REPRESENT THE EPITOME OF A DESIRED WALKING GAIT FOR A WALKING HORSE.* I find it quite interesting to note that many within the performance horse industry illustrate their most desired gait

as so laterally timed. Compare alignment of the performance horse weight bearing front leg with its hind leg furthest back and note how closely angles of these legs are aligned with almost identical slant. This indicates that the front leg is almost synchronized to the laterally paired hind. Isochronal timing, on the other hand is represented by the pleasure horse image where we see the hind supporting pair at their weight transfer point while the hooves of both front legs are arranged directly below the point of the shoulder, telling us that both front legs are shown mid stride, one

LIFT VS. PLACEMENT

Many people will talk about timing as one dimension of gait while never delving into it more than that. I stress both lift and placement when talking about timing because a hoof's liftoff can, and often does, have slightly different timing than its placement. "How can that be?" you ask. Compare the conformation of a horse's back legs to his front legs for the answer to this question.

Back legs and front legs have different jobs in carrying the horse. The front legs are more for weight bearing and less for forward thrust, while back legs are more suited to be the strong engine that pushes the horse directionally. Because their jobs are different these front and back legs have a different makeup and consequently travel differently. The front legs, with their knee bending action, have the ability to elevate their flight path into a higher arch as the horse uses his body to lighten the front by shifting some of the weight toward the rear. The horse needs this ability so he can climb uphill, jump over obstacles or for fighting, mating, etc. So his front legs can fold to lift as needed while the majority of the movement and effort of his back legs involves the hocks and stifles remaining closer to the ground and providing push for forward thrust. *The resulting arch of the front hooves compared to the sweeping action of the hind accounts for the back hooves' ability to maintain longer contact with the ground during a stride while the front hooves can have a greater non-weight bearing aerial phase.* Note that these differences are variable depending on how the horse is carrying himself and accounts for a slight difference of timing between lift and placement at many gaits.

Some people rely on the sound of the

weight bearing the other non-weight bearing. The alignment of the pleasure horse image represents true isochronal timing.

hoof beats to help determine the timing of the horse, but that method has its weakness because it only represents placement and does not reflect lift. We can listen to placement but it takes a practiced eye to see the lift off and determine the timing of that portion of this particular element. Both lift and placement are important in telling us how a horse is using his body and I assert that it is impossible to claim one is more definitive than the other.

Take the walking gaits in illustration. At the walk a horse's back hooves remain very close to the ground because it is a gait of non-suspension. However with increased speed and energy at the flatfoot walk and the running walk the front hooves tend to elevate from a little to a great deal more depending upon how much animation the horse is carrying. In the very animated walk where the headnod is reaching deep and prominent, and the front feet are marching with rhythmic purpose it is quite expected (even desired in show horses) to see great upward lift as well as forward reach and extension with those front legs. This greater reach, lift and even float of the front will all increase the aerial phase of the hooves with a higher arc while reducing the amount of time in contact with the ground. Greater float of the front end creates a significant and discernable difference of timing between lift and placement whenever it occurs at gait.

If you have a quality walking gait that has been polished and developed for an animated and showy walk, the increased action on the front can take an isochronal lift-off that supports that walk and morph it toward a slightly more diagonal placement. Many Walking Horse owners, trainers and even some judges might get concerned when a horse they had thought to be walking begins showing evidence of diagonal timing in the placement phase of their hooves only and consequently may begin to re-evaluate whether that horse might actually be foxtrotting instead. Let me state categorically that it takes much more to turn a walk into a foxtrot than a slight influence toward diagonal hoof placement, and anyone who doesn't realize this is doing both the walk and the foxtrot a tremendous disservice. There are many elements of gait, and the carriage of a horse cannot be labeled by only one of these elements, but rather needs to be judged as a whole. *This is why I stress the importance of watching lift off even more than placement when you're looking at walking gaits.* The lift gives a clearer picture of how the horse is actually using his body before the animation begins to influence his placement.

Often it is this difference in lift vs. placement timing that is the only thing breaking up an otherwise hard pace and morphing it into a stepping pace. Many performance horses are taught to travel in a pace through their posture and balance in preparation for carrying the additional weight and action devices, but then forced through framing into greater upward lift or jog on the front. This is an intentional and obvious mechanical delay being deliberately inserted into the gait by the rider. Anyone riding this way is forcing the horse away from a pure two beat hard pace illustrated by his liftoff timing, into a broken four-beat placement. There is a tremendous difference between a walk that starts and ends as a walk, and a stepping pace that begins as a pace. *A walk will be carried by the horse, so that he may be released*

into self carriage while traveling in that gear. However, a horse can never be released into gait while moving in the stepping pace that is being framed by the rider without immediately falling back into the hard two-beat pace. This is just one more reason why so many gaited horses are being constantly ridden with pressure on the bit and in their mouth.

You learn to see lift off better if you can closely watch the same-side pair of legs. I suggest watching the lateral pair of legs closest to you, keeping your eyes focused on the belly line of the horse while widening that focus to include the upper portion of that pair of legs in your view. This widening of focus takes a little practice, much like learning to see the 3-D Magic Eye puzzles by focusing beyond the level of the page. Focusing on the upper portion of the legs allows me to quickly determine if the back leg is breaking loose and starting its forward flight *before* the laterally paired front leg does. Further more in even timing the back hoof should not only lift off first, but should actually be halfway through its stride before the laterally paired front lifts off. It should have reached mid stride beneath the point of the hip which, at speed, gives the illusion that the back hoof almost bumps the front out of the way. You can practice seeing timing by watching video in the comfort of your living room. I actually recommend this since watching a video gives you the opportunity to stop the action in still frame and/or slow it down dramatically. Once you know what you're seeing you can speed it back up to practice at speed and train your eyes.

Speed

Speed is a variable of any gait or movement that horses carry. As a horse increases his speed eventually the nature of his gait will change, partly because speed is invariably accompanied by increased tension through their core. This increased tension changes the

way joints work; decreasing range of motion while adding support and power.

So exactly at what point does speed become definitive? When it changes the nature, appearance and function of the gait. The jogging trot of the western pleasure horse is very different from the extended trot often seen in a dressage ring. The shuffling stride of the saddle rack is likewise very different from the extended single-foot of the speed rack. Differences become even more definitive for the show ring. Judges are well-known for their desire to see an exhibitor demonstrate the range of style, ability and partnership with their horse by extending the speed of a desired gait, even when it may not be typically part of the gait calls for that particular class or exhibition.

This particular element can become confusing when it is the only difference between gait, much like we see with the walking gaits. The trail walk, ordinary walk, medium walk, flatfoot walk and running walk are all the same basic gait, with speed and its effects being the only difference. Note: the show walk of some open gaited rail classes is simply another way of calling for whatever walk is typically seen for your breed.

In the following pages we will address each of the primary easy gaits typically seen in the American gaited horse breeds and show you how these five *Elements of Gait* can illustrate the differences within the easy gaits, giving us quantifiable characteristics that make each of them identifiable. I also include additional tips to help you to quickly see a horse's gait. Once you understand them you will be able to watch for, learn to feel and finally to identify what gait your horse is doing.

Chapter 2 – Biomechanics of Easy Gaits

Biomechanics is the application of mechanical principles to a biological organism.

Biomechanics includes the study of the mechanical movement for any animal such as a horse. In this chapter I will use biomechanical principles to analyze the movement of gaited horse and how their biological attitude relates to their ability to carry their gaits.

I will explore each of five primary easy gaits most commonly seen in the American gaited horse breeds: flatfoot walk, running walk, foxtrot, stepping pace and the racking gaits. Utilizing the Elements of Gait previously outlined I will illustrate the definitive characteristics of each and give you an overview of the biomechanics involved. Much of your success with your own horse will likely depend on your understanding the correct movement for each gait as well as its commonly encountered faults.

THE WALKING GAITS

In most authoritative opinions a walk is ***the*** foundation gait for any horse. Until you get the walk established correctly it should continue to be your primary focus of training. The walk is an essential foundation for all gaited horses because it is the most relaxed, energy efficient AND THE MOST ISOCHRONALLY TIMED FOUR-BEAT GAIT. Every variation of walk should have distinct characteristics that are identifiable and consistent, and they are:

I have chosen to focus on these five primary gaits as most representative of those commonly encountered within the American gaited breeds. This is not to imply that other gaited horses will not benefit. In fact much of what I teach can and should be applied to any gaited horse, including those from South America, Iceland and elsewhere as well as grade or partially bred for gait. I have applied these same principles to many of these other breeds quite successfully. Their gaits are very similar or in many instances, the same with the only differences being more about terminology than anything else.

I will later address correction of common problem areas in the TRAINING CHAPTERS of this book. But felt that first you must understand WHAT SHOULD BE in order to comprehend where your own horse may be having difficulty and specifically what and how he needs to change to improve.

- Neutral core carried more level
- Even isochronal pick up *and* placement of each hoof
- Headnod working in time with the backend stride
- Non-suspended, both-hooves-on-the-ground weight transfer of both front and rear supporting leg pairs
- 3-2-3-2 hoof support sequence

I must stress how vital a relaxed and neutral topline is for a quality walking gait. It is this necessary neutral core that releases the spine so the horse may fluidly alternate dorsal, ventral and lateral muscle contractions. These muscles need to choreograph their contractions and releases in sequence to produce a four cornered, relaxed and energy efficient walking gait. Should any of them overwhelm or dominate this sequence it produces tension that eventually alters that gait. Tension is unavoidable when muscles contract in opposition to other contracting muscles. This alternating sequence must occur for a four beat gait, but when either the dorsal muscles overwhelm causing the spine to hollow, or the abdominal (ventral) muscles overwhelm to produce more roundness, these actions produce some unavoidable opposition of muscle contractions that creates added tension through the horse's core and causes the gait to alter. It is only in relaxed and neutral carriage that these tensions may be avoided to a greater degree.

In an overview, the fluid and alternating use of the core muscles enables the four cornered walking gaits to be executed with isochronal (even) timing. For a horse to walk with balanced and independent use of all four limbs he must have enough release throughout the topline to allow a moderate amount of both lateral bend as well as vertical rounding

and hollowing in alternating sequence. The lateral movement (side-to-side waggle) allows the legs to move closer together and further apart during each stride rotation, while the vertical hollowing and rounding assist in the pull and push movement of the legs.

I stated earlier how core muscle usage is key to independent leg movement, but it is important to note that the spine itself may also inhibit some fluid movement when a hollow topline occurs. The thoracic and lumbar vertebrae are shaped with spinous processes which is what we feel and sometimes see along the spine of a horse. These processes contract closer together when the back drops into hollow which actually helps support a weakening topline posture. The hollow attitude also increases stiffness that inhibits the lateral scissoring or waggle movement between front and hind legs, which consequently makes both isochronal and diagonal gaits more of an effort. While non-gaited horses can and often do travel in diagonal timing while carrying a hollow topline, the quality of that trot is almost always degraded and often out of sync. It is not unheard of for trotting breeds to actually find a lateral gait if the dorsal dominant core is severely hollow enough. This same hollow bracing through the core in the gaited horses makes it unlikely he can execute anything other than the laterally timed gait bred into their conformation.

AN ENERGY WAVE

It is the neutral topline and relaxed carriage through the core of a walking gait that allows the energy and drive of the hind limbs to flow through that core to be counterbalanced with the nodding of the head and neck. This is a highly visible characteristic of the flow of energy through the body when a horse is correctly executing a walking gait and though it is a signature of the walking and foxtrotting horses, it may be readily observed in almost every breed to a certain degree. The relaxed

topline allows this energy to flow uninhibited with what *FEELS LIKE* a wave of power emanating from the hindquarters and cresting toward the front. It becomes most visible in those horses with greater stride or who are executing a walk with stronger impulsion as when pulling heavy loads.

Lets breakdown specific movement to understand why we feel this wave of energy. The walks produce a seesaw movement as the shoulders lift and drop in alternating opposition to the lift and drop of the headnod. Why? Because the headnod is timed with his back legs which are in an opposite phase of stride than his front legs during isochronal timing. As the back hooves are both on the ground at their moment of weight transfer the shoulders are lifted with the front hooves both aligned directly below in mid-stride with one weight bearing, and one non-weight bearing. The head and poll drops to its lowest point while the back hooves are both on the ground. As the back stride moves to its midpoint with both hooves below the hip, the front hooves are reaching their moment of weight transfer allowing the shoulders to drop as the headnod lifts to its peak. This sequence creates a flow of energy or a wave that is established and driven by the back stride, flowing forward through the horse giving the rider the feel of riding a rolling wave. This is why the walking gaits are characterized by a softly rolling front to back motion of the saddle that coincides with the nodding of the head and the backend stride. *IF TENSION IN ANY FORM <u>AND AT ANY POINT</u> THROUGH THE TOPLINE INHIBITS THIS FLOW OF ENERGY THE GAIT WILL INEVITABLY CHANGE AWAY FROM A QUALITY WALK.*

There are many levelsor gears of walks that a horse can utilize, particularly gaited horses. While dressage requires as many as six speeds of walk, the gaited horses traditionally recognize three. I use an analogy of walking through the shopping mall to illustrate the different walking gaits. You have the window shopping speed of the trail walk; the I've-only-got-an-hour-to-make-it-to-both-stores speed of the flatfoot walk; and finally the hurrying I've-only-got-10-minutes-until-that-store-closes speed of the Running Walk. For the sake of this analogy we'll assume that we're not desperate enough to sprint through the mall. Since the trail walk is pretty standard among all breeds of horses, I'll not dwell on it here in any great depth, only to say that it's a relaxed isochronal walk with head lowered to its most relax position and the horse is moving with no hurry or sense of urgency at all.

FLATFOOT WALK

FLATFOOT WALK				
CORE POSTURE	HEAD & NECK ATTITUDE	WEIGHT TRANSFER / HOOF SUPPORT	TIMING	SPEED
Neutral - Level - Released	Loose - Level - Nodding Deap	No Suspension 2 - 3 - 2 - 3	Even - Isochronal	3 - 5 mph Marching Walk

Figure 2.1

When a horse is executing a bold flatfoot walk, I call it a deep walk because the horse reaches deep under himself in a sweeping stride while driving strong off his backend. This is a walk with purpose where the horse is moving like he has someplace to be. The tempo of the flatfoot walk stays moderate to slow, but the energy level and stride lengthen and *EXTENDS SUBSTANTIALLY* from the lower energy trail walk. The horse should be using himself with a neutral core while keeping the backend engaged so that he's *REALLY REACHING AND MAKING THE MOST OF EACH STRIDE*. There is no doubt to anyone watching this gait that the horse is moving *WITH PURPOSE* and not just moseyin' along. Remember the I've-only-got-an-hour analogy.

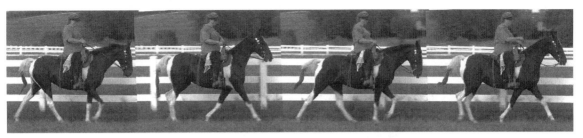

Figure 2.2 I'm Angle's Amazing Grace

What to look for:

The headnod becomes MOST PROMINENT and productive at this walking gait because the relaxed topline coupled with the slower tempo allows him to work his head and neck in deeper counter-balance to dramatically increase the energy of the backend stride. This counterbalanced weight adds power to the driving back end much like we swing our arms to counterbalance to our two foot stride, swinging more prominent as we walk faster. Consequently, when a horse is hooked up the bigger he strides the deeper the corresponding headnod. The headnodding action ORIGINATES FROM WITHIN THE SHOULDER with little movement of the poll itself. In other words there should be a stable angle that remains consistent between the head and the neckline, with all the up and down action originating from THE SHOULDER. Any flipping of the nose from the poll is unnecessary and could actually indicate the horse is trying to avoid lifting the frontend by utilizing a shallow head bob. Flipping the nose indicates poor use of balance and should be corrected by training a quiet head carriage willingly on the bit before you can begin to encourage correct lightness of the fore.

The driving engaged backend creates overstride, as the hind hoof sweeps well forward and overstrides" beyond the hoof print of the laterally paired fore that has just lifted off. Many believe the overstride measurement to be the most defining action of the flatfoot walk and running walk gaits, HOWEVER we will dispel this myth in great detail later in this book. Overstride at correct, isochronal timing may be anywhere from 6 to as much as 24 inches at the flatfoot walking speed. Less is acceptable as long as it does not indicate disengagement of the hind quarters. More overstride is acceptable AS LONG AS IT IS **NOT** A PRODUCT OF LATERAL TIMING. See the section titled **Overstride Illusion** in chapter 14 for more on this characteristic.

TRAINING THE FLATFOOT WALK

I recommend first getting your horse in sync with the tempo of your body; teaching them to rate their tempo and to follow your lead. Just as there can only be one leader in a dancing couple, the rider must lead and the horse must be willing to follow in this equitation partnership. If your horse is not willing to do this, then you need to work on this as part your contract with him. When a horse becomes responsive to your seat, legs and tempo it is time to begin asking them for more reach and more stride; to increase their energy WITHOUT INCREASING THEIR TEMPO. This is the single best tool to train a horse to extend any gait; communicating to him that you want bigger, not faster. Usually their initial response when you ask for more is to try giving you faster tempo with a shorter stride or to even break gait altogether. You must resist and correct any effort to lose form. Keep

By Anita J Howe

asking them to slow down the tempo and give you bigger stride with more reach. This is why it is so important to teach the horse to rate their tempo before moving on to this facet of the training.

This quote from Ray Hunt's **_THINK HARMONY WITH HORSES_**:

"A walk is a four beat gait and should be regular. You should be able to control it. If you want him to walk a little faster, you reach a little further with your legs, with your fanny, with the soles of your feet and the seat of your britches, with your MIND, with your positive thinking. You are picking his feet up and setting them down. You're going with him so he can learn to go with you – feel it. See how little it takes to do the job. If you can put your reins on the horn,

fold your arms and he will do it --- that's what you will do. Its feel, timing and balance. It can become as natural as breathing

When the horse really strides out and engages his energy at this slower tempo flatfoot walk it will produce that thump-thump-thump-thump sound that characterizes the flatfoot walk. The sound is produced as each hoof lands flat at a prominent marching speed, and is where the name flatfoot walk originates. It's exciting when you hear this signature sound and know your horse is really working the gait well.

For more training advice on the flatfoot walk see the chapter 15 for training the naturally brilliant walking gaits.

COMMON PROBLEMS

It is critical to understand that your horse CAN walk shallow and you need to learn to feel this. By shallow I mean that he can disengage his hindquarters, adding tension to his hips, shortening his stride and start jigging or suspending with his backend weight transfer. I'm *NOT* talking about a foxtrot which many may disparagingly call it. This is a fault that is more about engagement and proper use of the hindquarters, not timing. I've heard the term *dinkers* applied, and wish folks understood how easy it is to correct this when you learn to feel it. Disengagement comes from overriding the walking speed a horse is comfortable with and not correcting him when it happens. As you push for increased energy and speed without having the understanding or feel to realize when your horse begins to shorten their stride, you are setting yourself up for this common gait fault. Though it's not critical for pleasure riders it does start them on the pathway toward an off-gait, and becomes that first nudge away from true isochronal timing. The less engaged the backend the easier it is for a horse to lose form and when that happens you'll be lucky to end up with a

rack (at least the rack is still smooth to ride), but all too often you end up with either pace or trot. So pay attention, watch and feel for it. Bump and release your horse (I recommend a one-rein half-halt discussed later), slowing him until you feel his hips release, his backend settle and his stride lengthen. Be persistent and insist on this engagement. Don't allow him to go shallow or uncorrected if you want to develop more a brilliant intermediate speed in correct form.

Disengagement can also be caused by *HOW* we ask for the increase of speed and energy. Remember that when you're ready to transition up to the flatfoot walk from the slower trail walk you should do so very subtly with a driving seat. Lean forward very slightly into a three-point seat while draping your legs backward a very moderate amount; just enough to show the horse you are eager. Some horses are so sensitive to leg cues that this is all it takes. Sometimes a soft cluck along with an increase of your movement in the saddle is sufficient to encourage him to pick up his energy. *IF YOU ARE ABRUPT IN YOUR CUE TO SPEED UP IT IS QUITE NATURAL FOR YOUR HORSE TO THINK*

YOU WANT A <u>DIFFERENT GEAR</u>. We need to keep things understated and a little more gradual so that he will begin to realize we want increased energy while remaining in the same gear. We want him *to "rev his engine, <u>not</u> change his gears".* Note this same method should be used with Walking Horses training the running walk from the flatfoot walk. Be subtle so he will stay in the same form and just increase his energy, reach and tempo.

"If he ain't noddin', he ain't walkin'!" I'm certain most of you have heard this saying at some point. It's completely accurate; much more so than many in the modern Walking Horse industry would like to admit, and it amazes me sometimes how few horses consistently winning in some TWH show circuits have so little true headnod and still win. The movement or usage of the head and neck are a product of what is happening with everything behind. *HEADNOD DOES NOT CREATE GAIT BUT IS AN EXPRESSION OF WHAT GAIT IS BEING CARRIED* and as such tells its tale.

The biomechanics of the flatfoot walk promote a headnodding counterbalanced action that should be at *ITS MOST PROMINENT* in this gait. Where you lose the headnod is most often due to tension through the topline… oftentimes this is because the horse is moving away from the true isochronal timing, but sometimes a lack of balance and conditioning will predispose a horse to increase tension for support. Horses carrying themselves heavy on the fore are notorious for losing the quality nodding head of the walking gait because the headnod is aided by lightness on the front. Poor fitting saddles; harsh bitting causing a horse to evade contact; even conformational issues can all result in added topline tension that will compromise his ability to release and nod his head productively. Whatever the reason, if your horse is not nodding correctly, I recommend examining some of these potential issues. Not just because of gait quality, but in concern for his comfort and longevity as a pleasure horse.

Speed is the final common fault found at the flatfoot walk. Form should never be sacrificed for increased speed. This statement is consistent in almost every rule book in the country that I'm familiar with. While it's not as critical to the pleasure rider, it does become more of an issue for those wishing to exhibit.

- Many riders mistakenly override their horse at slow-to-moderate running walk speeds when they think they are in the flatfoot walk and end up losing its unique characteristics. The two primary distinctions between the flatfoot walk and the running walk are the deep nodding head (which becomes more shallow at the increased tempo of the running walk) just as the flatfoot placement becomes more rolling (heel-to-toe) as the horse increases its speed. We will soon discuss the running walk, but suffice to say that if you push into the running walk speeds when the flatfoot walk is called for, you will have nowhere to go *AND STILL MAINTAIN FORM* when the running walk is finally called.

- Many people claim that length of stride and overstride should both have greater extension at the running walk. When the running walk is built correctly from the flatfoot walk this is indeed correct, but my only concern with this statement is that they then fail to properly develop the flatfoot walk to its greatest potential. I recommend not getting too caught up in this aspect of the running walk until it is well established and polished. Your first priority should be extending the reach of the flatfoot walk at a slower tempo which then allows your horse to show a definitive increase when transitioning to his intermediate gait. By developing the length of stride at the slower tempo flatfoot walk you may easily accomplish a 4 -5 mph speed, as the extended stride adds brilliance to this foundation gait. From this well established flatfoot walk you have a wonderful foundation to bring on a solidly extended running walk.

For more training tips on the walking gaits see Part IV <u>*Developing the Naturally Brilliant Walking Horse*</u>

Consistent speed in the show ring is another commonly encountered problem, but not really of much concern to the pleasure rider. I often see horses under-ridden in speed, dropping down into trail walk gear. The energy is not as bold and purposeful at the trail walk, and the headnod is less prominent. To me this is a more forgivable mistake and easily corrected by asking for a little more energy. Many overridden horses have really never been trained to find the bold, high energy and slower tempo flatfoot walk, and that is truly a shame for it can be a very brilliant and showy gait.

So how did we seem to lose the flatfoot walk? Is it a result of wanting the get the gait too quickly? Are we so eager to get a running walk that we just sort of slide right past the flatfoot walk? Maybe it's from the influence of performance horse training and competitions where young colts are deliberately pushed for speed in order to add pace and swing to their gait. Wherever we lost it, we need to find it and bring it back. *THE FLATFOOT WALK IS THE FOUNDATION GAIT FOR MOST GAITED BREEDS*, and so essential that I believe all young horses should be flatfoot walked, almost exclusively, *FOR THEIR FIRST YEAR UNDER SADDLE*, especially if you have intentions of showing them eventually. Good muscle development at this gait and posture will make the running walk and any of the intermediate gaits even better and easier for the horse. The benefits are numerous:

- A well executed flatfoot walk, engaging the correct frame and carriage will be the most evenly timed gait. Once it's well established, this timing will naturally want to carry forward as the horse increases its speed will help avoid the horse from defaulting to a trot or pace as you ask them to find an speedier intermediate gait.

- For Walking Horses, bigger stride and reach can be developed at the flatfoot walk better than at any other speed, particularly with those that don't really want to stride out for you. It's quite natural for horses to want to shorten their stride as they increase their tempo and speed. If you desire more stride extension then the flatfoot walk is the gait to train and condition for it. Remember to ask your horse for *bigger, not faster.*

- Working at the flatfoot walk is the single best natural horsemanship tool to correct off-gaited horses, those horses that DO want to fall toward the trot or pace and lose that smooth riding four-beat. A good flatfoot walk will teach, develop and cement the correct form, carriage and muscle memory for what will later become a natural and effortless four-beat intermediate gait.

- The flatfoot walk is an easy and pleasurable gait for the horse while still efficiently covering a lot of ground. A 3-5 mph flatfoot walk will normally outdistance other breeds out on the trail while not overly tiring horse or rider. These horses, like the Energizer Bunny, just keep going and going...

- A nice slower tempo at the flatfoot walk will then provide a more dramatic increase in speed when the running walk is asked for in the show ring; just remember *to keep the energy, stride and headnod big*, while asking for that slower tempo.

I want to encourage everyone to focus on this gait and give it the importance that it deserves in developing their gaited horses. I would like to someday see all show classes for young gaited horses (4yrs and under) require only a trail walk and a flatfoot walk, and save that speedier intermediate gaits for the mature horses. This gait is that important. Everything else is built upon it; the coordination and muscles take time for many of these horses to develop. In order to do it faster they must first do it right, and your horse is worth the investment.

THE RUNNING WALK

RUNNING WALK				
CORE POSTURE	HEAD & NECK ATTITUDE	WEIGHT TRANSFER / HOOF SUPPORT	TIMING	SPEED
Neutral - Level - Released	Loose - Level - Nodding Shallow	No Suspension 2 - 3 - 2 - 3	Even - Isochronal	6 - 10 mph Rolling Walk

Figure 2.3

The running walk is the same fundamental gear as the flatfoot walk, carried with increased tempo, speed and often added extension. The core posture remains neutral or level while the croup will coil with the beginnings of collection to support the increased backend drive. A horse should exhibit lightness in the front aided by this total engagement and drive from a driving backend which allows them to continue rolling loosely and freely out of their shoulders. The back hooves drive with power and strength, consistently overstriding the track of the laterally paired front hoof.

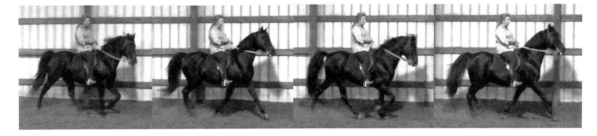

Figure 2.4 Papa's Royal Delight

The neutral topline keeps the timing even and isochronal, though it is not uncommon to feel some increased tension through the core as the horse increases his speed. Inherent with any gait increased speed promotes an increase of tension. *PLEASE NOTE* however, that proper conditioning of a correct running walk along with a solid foundation of a strong flatfoot walk enables horses to carry the greater speed with less tension and thereby develop a more energy efficient running walk. This fluid and energy efficient gait was the overriding purpose of foundation breeding for the Tennessee Walking Horse. Their need was for a utility mount that could cover many miles comfortably and reliably. Less topline tension will also tend to produce more brilliance in this natural gait. Where many exhibitors go wrong is their attempt to artificially enhance the running walk with mechanics or by adding weight to the front hooves. We discuss this in great detail in my final chapter dealing with the performance horse training.

The running walk stride will often extend beyond the length seen at the flatfoot walk, but not always. While extended stride and reach is very desirable, the running walk does not always produce an increase of these *IF* the flatfoot walk is properly trained and conditioned to maximize both. It is my experience that tremendous extension of stride can be achieved at the flatfoot walk, and that horses with this conditioning can be quite brilliant in their running walk as well as maintain better form while increasing their speed and tempo. Because they have this remarkable extension at the flatfoot walk, you will often see the stride length remain consistent as tempo and speed increases. Because stride is a key component in a gait's efficiency any reduction with increased speed indicates a need for further training and conditioning. If a rider is unable to feel the stride of their horse, it is not uncommon to see a shortening of stride in horses pushed too quickly for speed before their conditioning is ready to carry it.

Just like the flatfoot walk, the headnod is vital for a correct running walk. Show ring practices aside, the old saying of "if he ain't noddin', he ain't walkin'" is still worth carving into stone for the headnod is the single best indicator that the horse is maintaining his neutral topline and desired looseness, as well as his non-suspended weight transfer. What you will see as a flatfoot walk transitions to the running walk is a productive headnod becoming slightly more shallow as the tempo increase. Simply put the horse does not have the time to drop as deeply in the headnod at the faster tempo running walk. Also, as much as we desire the horse to maintain looseness, there

will invariably be some increase in tension (less is better) due to the increase in speed, going back to the rule of biomechanics that states that any extension of speed creates an increase in muscle tension. The more we condition and encourage our horse to retain his released topline the more energy efficient and brilliant the running walk will be. Though we train for less tension, more looseness and release, we must realize that some is unavoidable. Don't blame your horse, just patiently keep working and asking for release. As his core and haunch muscles become stronger the speed will become easier to bring on while retaining true looseness and brilliance.

The running walk is an intermediate gait whose speed should comfortably extend from 6-9 mph. Many claim to have horses that carry a faster running walk, but it is my experience that most, if not all, of these horses that are reputed to carry double-digit speeds are actually carrying more of a racking-walk or a stepped pace when you carefully study their form. Some are even moving toward a flying pace at their top speeds. It is both the neutral topline and the loose, relaxed carriage that enable a horse to maintain true isochronal timing and correct form while increasing their speed. As stated earlier, the greater the speed the greater the propensity for tension through the body. The greater the tension the more likely it will alter the horse's form away from a desirable isochronal timing toward either end of the gait spectrum; the pace or the trot depending on the proclivities of your horse.

Those horses that have learned to maintain the even timing as they gain speed have the best opportunity to find a fluid running walk without losing form. However even isochronal timing cannot prevent a loss of form. A correct running walk at its top speed will naturally morph into an off-gait if pushed beyond that natural limit that the horse has been conditioned to carry. Because a walk is defined as a gait with weight transfer occurring between hooves that are both in contact with the ground (non-suspended), it is rare indeed to see any horse that can maintain this critical characteristic while increasing speed much into double digits. Rare indeed are the horses that can execute correct form of the running walk above 10-11 mph speeds. I am not saying that no horses can accomplish this just that they are few and far between and most likely well over 16 hands in height.

Is it really a walk?

It is worth note that the only exception to the walking 3-2-3-2 hoof support that I am aware of is during some running walks when horses will exhibit strong enough backend engagement and drive with light croup collection to create a *NATURAL* float or suspension on of the front half of their bodies. You can find horses that have enough natural lift *THROUGH THEIR CORE FROM A STRONG BACKEND* to maintain the loose rolling reach of the walking shoulder. This *natural float* then creates the only exception I know of to that 3 – 2 – 3 – 2 correct walking support sequence, morphing it into a 3 – 2 – 1 – 2 – 3 – 2 – 1 – 2 sequence of support as the floating front results in a *VERY MINUTE* single hoof support for each of the back hooves.

This is not to be confused with when horses are actually carrying a racking movement with their shoulders braced for a *SIGNIFICANT* aerial phase of suspension during the weight transfer between those front hooves. *THIS* action is frequently rewarded as desirable in the performance show rings. However several judging associations will correctly penalize horses that have this exaggerated lift and break at the knee *WITHOUT EQUIVALENT REACH*. When a horse braces his shoulders for exaggerated lift, he will quite naturally reduce his forward reach and his headnod will become barely discernable, even non-existent. This produces a bicycling or jogging movement with the front end. The horse has ceased walking with

There are limits to this gait while maintaining form and it becomes a reality of physics on how much speed can be accomplished while maintaining the both-hooves-on-the-ground weight transfer. Much like humans can never speed walk as fast as they can sprint no matter how long they condition themselves. If your horse has a solidly isochronal walking gait he will likely morph to an evenly timed rack at the upper reaches of his speed.

his front pair of supporting legs. It is the notable lack of roll and forward reach through the shoulder that is the principal difference in the two examples I've described here. In the first, the horse is still carrying a walk with roll and reach on his front end complete with productive headnod working off the backend stride. It is also supported by the suspension coming from a strong core that floats his front. In the second example braced shoulders have inherently changed how the horse is using the front of his body, as signified by the jogging front legs and the total lack or severe reduction of headnod.

Many will argue that the float action also disqualifies the gait as a true walking gait. I've heard others argue that all running walks will have this slight to exaggerated suspension in the front in attempt to defend the practice of rewarding the racking-walk (a.k.a. the single-foot walk) of the performance trained show horses. However I know this particular claim to be false for I've personally worked with many western and trail pleasure going horses that carry a lower headset with level front-to-back balance that roll and reach equally with the front and the rear legs even at extended speeds. Indeed, this level balance executed with a true 3 – 2 – 3 – 2 hoof support is much more energy efficient in my mind, and more in line with the purpose of the foundation breeding.

I personally feel that the truth lay in

between, with a very fine line of separation. The natural float of a horse that has developed extreme engagement and strong conditioning of the backend can produce a very brilliant and showy gait that I find very compelling. Much as the natural lift of upper dressage movements are to be admired. *IF* the movement comes from the strength and conditioning of the backend with a strongly coiled loin and is **not** a product of any extreme modifications, absurd training techniques or mechanical manipulations, it is a truly a thing of beauty. Naturally brilliant float is easy to identify and differentiate from the mechanized and artificially trained gait in that it maintains a rolling and reaching shoulder with productive headnod, while the mechanically trained, artificial gait will tend to lose this natural brilliance as the horse sacrifices forward roll and reach for a bicycling, knee breaking up-and-down jog. Once you see the float you KNOW it's a natural, fluid and brilliant gait that has nothing to do with what's on the horse feet. He should be able to carry this natural float just as easily barefoot as shod because it comes from a well conditioned backend.

FEEL FROM THE SADDLE

From the saddle there are two distinct sensations experienced by the rider in the running walk. First is that this gait IS an extension of the other walking gaits and as such will have the same flow or wave of energy emanating from the backend through the same neutral topline carriage and expressed through the headnod of the horse. The difference is that as your horse increases both tempo and speed there will be some added essential tension through his core. What is crucial to note here is that the better quality, more brilliantly natural running walk will maintain a high degree of relaxed neutral core and the increased tension will focus on the coiling of the loins rather than in the core itself. The ability to carry faster and faster speed at the running walk is conditioned and built as the horse advances in training. Building the gait from a flatfoot walk is highly recommended to maintain correct, even timing. My experience is that a horse continues to improve his running walk year after year in both stride and speed. So don't be overly concerned if you're not able to get much beyond a 7-8 mph gait in the early years. Patience and consistent riding will help your horse continue to bring on his speed with each year.

It is unavoidable that faster tempo will equal more compact movement in the rolling headnod. The headnod should still be undeniably evident but due to his faster up and down movement remaining in time to his driving backend stride that has also sped up, the head and neck simply do not have the time to dip as deeply at the running walk. While the speedier tempo shortens the headnod, consequently the front-to-back rolling motion of the saddle will quiet and become more compact as well, so that many feel the running walk to be even smoother than the flatfoot walk to ride.

The next sensation of note in the running walk is the lightness that should be maintained from the saddle forward. While increasing his energy and drive a horse needs to lighten on this fore to avoid becoming heavy in front. The proper balance for a running walk should always be built upon backend engagement and drive. If you feel your horse getting heavier toward the fore as you increase his speed, be cautious that he is likely flirting with fore-heavy foxtrot and you will need to correct this before allowing him to move faster.

A great running walk should be built from an excellent flatfoot walk. The flatfoot walk is the foundation and the running walk can only develop from a properly balance slower gait.

I know many in the traditional performance show world still train the running walk *by taking a hold of* the pace and framing a vertical face to break up the two beat pacing gait. But the reality is that this method is neither correct training practice nor produces correct

gait. You **will** get a gait, but it will not be a fluid and correctly balanced running walk and will obviously lack self carriage by the horse. Of further consideration is the risk of actually causing your horse to become more unbalanced rather than helping.

THE STEPPING PACE

STEPPING PACE [AMBLE]				
CORE POSTURE	HEAD & NECK ATTITUDE	WEIGHT TRANSFER / HOOF SUPPORT	TIMING	SPEED
Dorsal Dominant - Hollow	Higher & Mostly Fixed	Front Suspension None Behind 3 - 2 - 1 - 2 - 3	Lateral - Broken Pace	8 - 12 mph

Figure 2.5

A.k.a. Step-and-pace, step-pace or stepped pace. However you label it in your region this gait is a very laterally timed, four-beat gait where the thoracolumbar core is most often in a moderately to extremely hollow carriage and exhibiting tremendous dorsal muscle dominance. The croup, however, will often remain coiled keeping the backend stride sweeping with *walking* engagement. Most often there is very little headnod due to the added tension throughout the horse's body. This tension through the core inhibits the ability to counterbalance the use of the head and neck to that backend stride. In effect it blocks the energy flow from the sweeping backend stride and short circuits the *expression* of the stride through the front of the horse.

Core tension along with a hollow topline alignment demonstrate a horse that is actually in more of a pacing frame where the pace is being broken up by over flexion forced and framing of the head. While not always the case, in a majority of horses some pressure is constantly maintained through the bit to

assist in squaring up this lateral carriage. I've even heard several trainers try to explain to me how *"gaited horses can't really gait without pressure in the mouth."* Huh?

There are some horses that do naturally carry their intermediate gait with some essential tension through their core and a moderately hollow posture. This carriage often produces a side to side lateral motion through their body. It is not unusual to sometimes see this side to side counterbalancing movement expressed through the head and neck in offset to the body's motion. These horses have learned to carry a smooth pleasure gait, without completely unlocking their core into totally independent four cornered looseness and movement. I see this with horses that are a little more nervous in temperament and ones that tend to balance a little heavier forward. It often takes only a little bit training with some bending and softening to teach them to relax and release. The real patience and persistence is needed in teaching them to maintain that looseness while they increase energy and speed since both speed and energy expansion naturally trigger an increase of core tension.

Many riders honestly prefer this laterally timed gait for its natural speed potential. While it is not as energy efficient as the running walk, the stepping pace can carry

FEEL FROM THE SADDLE

When a horse is lifted and light through his lower neck and wither, and soft on the bit the stepping pace can be one of, if not THE smoothest gait to ride because it has none of the front-to-back movement of the running walk and is broken just far enough from the pace to seriously reduce any side-to-side motion supported by that gait. You get the benefit of great speed and forward boost supported by the lateral timing and it is almost as addictive to ride as the racking gaits often are when carried by a horse with strong backend engagement and frontend lightness.

However if a horse is seriously overloaded onto his fore, the stepping pace ride often becomes very rough as his front hooves feel as though they almost jam into the ground producing a rather abruptly jarring ride. The

IS IT A PACE?

More frequent still are those horses that *truly are* traveling in a totally lateral pace where the rider is tightly framing the bit in attempt to mechanically square them into gait. The lower neck becomes seriously dropped during

more forward speed with its laterally timed swing. Many trail riders and aficionados of field trial competitions particularly like both the stepping pace and the lateral rack for both comfort to the rider and speed at gait.

fore-heavy horse is also lacking in lightness an the ride is not only uncomfortable but can be taxing to the horse's frame. Overall the heavy on the fore stepping pace is not a good posture for a horse to carry a rider long term. This unbalanced stepping pace is frequently seen in young horses that are started far too early in life and simply do not have the strength in their topline to support the weight of the rider while remaining neutral and in balance. It is also seen in mature horses that have been ridden braced on the bit for many years. If your horse is carrying himself in a stepped pace gait that feels very uncomfortable to ride, please see the exercises in the training section of this book on helping your horse rebalance, lighten his fore and soften his core muscles. You and your horse will be happier.

the step pace or pace and all pressure on the bit shortens the neckline, exerting pressure on the downward "S" curve of the cervical vertebrae.

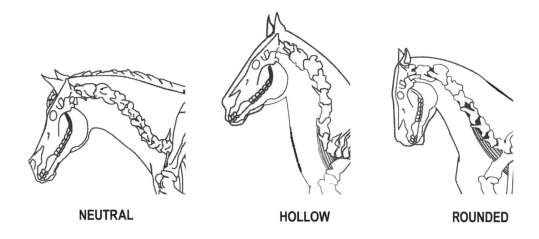

NEUTRAL   HOLLOW   ROUNDED

Cervical Vertebrae - Lift at the lower neck

Figure 2.6

This downward pressure inhibits the horse's ability to lift and lighten this lower neck thereby locking the horse into a rigidly braced shoulder and neck carriage. It is therefore very common to feel these horses tending to lean into the bit as they move heavier on the fore and often stumble over uneven ground from their inability to stride lightly on the front. Lacking the essential lift of the lower neck promotes a ***catch 22*** prompting the rider to attempt forcibly lifting the horse specifically to encourage lightness but in reality making this condition more exaggerated. The ante gets upped by increasing pressure and using longer shank until the flexion becomes even more severe, the lower neck more blocked. The unfortunate by-product of this type of riding is a horse that becomes more and more uncomfortable, locked up and unbalanced leaning heavily into rather severe bitting. Sometimes the pressure on the bit becomes so extreme that physical damage may be caused to the tissues of the mouth.

Eventually, if the rider is both persistent and insistent the horse may resolve to find a knee-jogging upward action with his front knees and fetlocks that will break up the two-beat pace into a barely broken four-beat stepping pace. This jogging action reduces forward reach while it increases both lift and break. While mechanically breaking up a pace produces a smoother ride, you can often note that these horses appear unhappy and uncomfortable. Their frame is often so hollow and locked that ventral muscles may very well begin to atrophy as the dorsal muscling becomes stronger and more dominant. These hollow and pacing horses become so acclimated to traveling in this manner they require patient re-conditioning to unlock their frame or their orthopedic soundness may well decline after years of carrying this posture. Dressage instructors have been known to refer to these horses as "*broken in half*" because the topline is so dropped into hollow as the rider desperately pulls on the bit trying to rebalance a heavy on the fore horse. The truly sad part of this situation is both the discomfort being experienced by the horse and the fact that all this misguided effort of the rider can, and often does, make it worse instead of helping.

Higher head carriage and a downward lock lower neck both encourage a nosed-out face, so severe bitting with seriously long shanks are often used to overcome that tendency and force a more vertical head-set. ***Please note***

that headset is NOT head carriage, nor is it collection. The defining difference is that a head-set is a framed, forced and held-in posture much like Rollkur, while head carriage is something offered by the horse and maintained on a loose or light rein. Collection is for another chapter entirely and has very little to do with the head.

Many performance trainers admire this highly framed head carriage and actually promote this style of gait. Carried to the extreme it becomes a knee-bending, chest-thumping bicycle action admired and often rewarded in the ring. You can understand therefore how this method has evolved into the traditional way to alter a completely lateral pacing gait to break it up into a stepping pace. It requires little training of the horse, just persistent *"collect 'em up"* mentality and force from the rider, and/or mechanical intervention of the farrier. Both the core posture and the laterally paired lift-off label it a pacing gait while the placement becomes a smoother four beat ride.

If you're unable to determine if a horse is doing a running walk or a stepping pace study the lift-off of the lateral pairs. This is easier once you train your eyes to focus above the knees and hocks. You should be able to see the back leg break loose first, starting its forward aerial sweep a half step ahead of the laterally paired front hoof. If you cannot see this back hoof starting forward ahead of the front and

these legs appear to be synchronized then as far as the horse's posture is concerned he's still executing a pace, even if the front snap is breaking up into four beats. If you want an isochronally timed gait then you must train for it, not simply override the horse into a pace then take a hold of him to frame up a smooth ride. If you wish to ride a stepping pace then by all means do so, but be aware that you should alternate gaits to allow your horse to release the dorsal dominant posture periodically to aid his continued orthopedic soundness. Further, I cannot recommend riding the stepping pace too much if you hope to eventually train a slow rolling canter as the posture of the two gaits are not compatible.

I would further advise that even for those who like the forward speed of the stepping pace, some softening and bending exercises will help your horse rebalance and greatly benefit his topline. As I frequently see in training those breeds that have a signature gait more in line with a stepping pace, such as the Mountain Horses and Icelandics, softening of core muscles, added lightness in the fore and bit training all contribute to produce a much more relaxed self carriage and overall happier horse. Far too many horses are not as balanced, and need constant support through the bit or will again fall heavy on the fore. This less than ideal carriage is really very easy to correct with a little patient effort and training.

THE FOXTROT (FOX TROT)

FOXTROT				
CORE POSTURE	HEAD & NECK ATTITUDE	WEIGHT TRANSFER / HOOF SUPPORT	TIMING	SPEED
Ventral Dominant - Rounded	Level to Low - Shallow Nod	Back Suspension None in Front 3-2-1-2-3	Diagonal - Broken Trot	6 - 9 mph

Figure 2.7

The foxtrot is a moderate speed, broken diagonal intermediate gait. It is one where the natural balance of the horse is carried more toward the fore with those front legs reaching in a both-hooves-on-the-ground walking weight transfer coupled with a jogging, lightly disengaged backend that exhibits a very brief moment of suspension during its weight transfer. The topline is usually carried between neutral to round, and is unique in that the core is actually more rounded than the croup. The loins of the croup are often somewhat uncoiled as they lighten into a jogging stride. There is a moderate amount of tension through the hips to support that jogging backend while the head and neck are often level, even low. Both the hip tension and the shortened rear stride reduce the depth and counterbalance of the nodding head from that of the flatfoot walk. This shortened headnod exhibits more action at the poll and less from the shoulder as opposed to the deep and consistent nod of the walking gaits.

The Foxtrot is a gait that many stock-type horses can even be taught to find. These soft trotters were always prized by ranchers and cowboys as premier working horses. The foxtrot takes the normal up and down jog of the trot and smoothes it into a front-to-back push or jig that enables the rider to support their weight on their seat without losing saddle contact. There is no upward lofting, just a pushing front-to-back. While it may not sound like a huge difference to some, when you spend many hours in the saddle this becomes *quite* significant. It is very energy efficient for the horse because the walking carriage of the fore prevents the majority of their weight (and yours) from being lofted upward.

While some overstride is acceptable or even desired in the show ring it is the surefooted stride of the gait that is so very desirable to many who pleasure ride this gait.

The Fox Trotting horse breed that was founded in the Ozark Mountains of Missouri where a sturdy and sure footed gait was highly prized. While the registry remained "open" many walking horses were cross-registered upon exhibiting an ability to carry this unique gait. In general, the breed exhibits a slightly shorter stride than many Walking Horses, producing a more stable and sure-footed carriage at this broken diagonal gait. The surefooted carriage makes them a gaited breed imminently suitable for rugged and mountainous terrain. While the more laterally timed gaits tend to promote a more forward movement and can be carried at greater speed, the more level and rounded topline of the foxtrot lends itself to a more balanced gait. This posture also allows the horse to carry a lower head for better scrutiny of possible obstacles and more secure hoof placement and balance over rough terrain.

Don't be misguided into thinking that only Missouri Foxtrotters perform the foxtrot. Like most American gaited breeds, these horses are all very multi-gaited and can just as often be seen executing a stepping pace, a saddle rack or even a very fluid running walk as they are a foxtrot. So too can many gaited breeds can be trained to find a variety of gaits, *INCLUDING THE FOXTROT* when they learn to unlock their core, changing their posture and balance. As we've discussed, these are key elements to opening a horse to a wide range of his gaiting potential. Most pleasure riders are content to allow their horse to settle into whatever gait they are happy with as long as it's a smooth ride, and they are willing to carry that gait indefinitely.

From the saddle the foxtrot gait is a natural progression for many horses from the flatfoot walk if they have an easy ability to round up through their core and have not had the training to rebalance themselves to maintain hindquarter engagement. The progression from flatfoot walk to the foxtrot usually happens backend first. In other words the increasing energy at the flatfoot walk makes a transition into the foxtrot by lightening the backend slightly ahead of the fore. In many untrained horses the foxtrot tends to be a narrow corridor of gait found briefly during transition between the flatfoot walk and the hard trot. By slowing that transition, and *CAREFULLY BUILDING THE ENERGY* of the flatfoot walk while keeping the head and neck moderately low, you will help your horse to not pass right through this sturdy and surefooted easy gait. Care should be taken not to allow the speed to overtake the horse's carriage or you will find yourself riding a fully diagonal hard trot in a heartbeat. The foxtrot is just shy of the hard trot, with just enough broken diagonal timing to smooth out the ride. Many riders do not recognize it as a legitimate gait at first, thinking it is just a phase of transition. Often you may find at that moment of foxtrot (or transition) quick, light bit contact (not enough to dramatically change head position) can slow or stop the transition and enable the horse to remain in this gait longer. Persistent riding will soon have him working comfortably at the foxtrot for longer and longer periods. When a horse recognizes that you desire him to remain in this gait, most are quite willing and happy to do so. Upon establishing this gear, you can then begin to condition a horse to slowly extend his speed while remaining in this effortless easy gait.

While I am not opposed to utilizing a light, brief bit connection to tell the horse to slow or stop his transition, I am opposed to any kind of constant bit contact that braces the horse's head into position or frames into a gait and I highly encourage riders to release their horse once they've gotten found the desired gear and only correct him as he begins to shift away from what is most desired. It is this release that encourages him to remain in gait, improving self carriage as well as teaching him that it *is* the desired gait.

Common faults at the Foxtrot:
• Overriding the 5-8 mph speed of the

gait before the horse is conditioned and sliding into a hard 2 beat trot.
• Another commonly seen problem is throwing the head high and hollowing into the pace. This problem is due to the forward balance of the foxtrot transitioning easily into a forward balanced stepping pace or hard pace with just a simple hollowing of his core. This can also be a result of back discomfort causing a resistant frame.
• Bracing from bit evasion causing the horse to hold his head fixed and morphing into a fox-rack (broken diagonal racking gait), or the more common off-gait of the pace. Most pleasure riders will not differentiate between a fox-rack and a foxtrot, defining the gait only from the similar timing of the lift and placement of the hooves. Both are carried with slight forward balance, both have a suspended backend weight transfer and both have broken diagonal timing. The fox-rack is differentiated by its suspended weight transfer *ON THE FORE AS WELL AS THE HIND*. Like all the racking gait variations, it involves suspended weight transfer of both supporting pairs, producing the 2-1-2-1 hoof support sequence of the rack. Further, when the horse begins suspending on the front he further loses the headnod that characterizes the foxtrot. The bracing of the shoulders for suspension blocks the energy of the back stride from flowing through to counter-balance with a nodding head.

Training for a foxtrot should always progress from the flatfoot walk. I recommend asking the horse to subtly increase his energy output while carrying a moderately level head carriage. At first it will feel like a light jig on the backend of the walk and this is the gear you need to encourage in your horse to build and reinforce this as a gait to him. He will most likely think he's in between gears, and a very light check-and-release when you feel the gait will reinforce it and tell him you wish him to stay there. If he still insists on continuing to the hard trot, I use a one-rein half-halt to bend him slightly to resist his inclination to continue that progression, followed by a release as soon as he settles back into gait. If he refuses to listen to the half-halt, you must bring him back to the flatfoot walk and start building your progression again.

Some riders and trainers find it beneficial to support the horse in his gait by making bit contact just as he moves up into the foxtrot and maintaining a supporting rein the entire time

he is carrying the gait. I can see how this might be helpful to keep him in gait, but it will not teach the horse self-carriage at that gait. Plus I personally object to any gait needing constant bit contact for support because it is too easy for this contact to become unintentionally abusive if great care is not taken. I prefer to train the horse to carry the gait without maintaining the anchor of bit contact promoted by many. If any horse is giving me the gait I want I believe he deserves to have the freedom of his head, especially if that gait requires some headnodding movement.

FEEL FROM THE SADDLE

The foxtrot produces an abbreviated, front-to-back jig that can be quite easy on the rider because the seat never lofts upward, away from the saddle. Because of the broken diagonal timing the forward speed will be slightly more limited to a 5-8 mph intermediate

speed. However, many Foxtrotters trained for the show ring have learned to extend their stride, reach and speed. This could account for a greater degree of movement in the saddle frequently seen in the foxtrotting show horses.

THE RACKING GAITS

RACKING GAITS				
CORE POSTURE	HEAD & NECK ATTITUDE	WEIGHT TRANSFER / HOOF SUPPORT	TIMING	SPEED
Rigid - Dorsal Dominant to Level	Higher & Fixed	Full Suspension Front and Back 2-1-2-1-2	Even to Lateral	6 mph Shuffle to 30 mph Speed Rack

Figure 2.8

The racking gaits have a huge range of both speed and form, all carried with the same tightly held tension through the core, high fixed head carriage, with suspended weight transfer and a hoof support sequence of 2-1-2-1-2-1. The variations happen with both timing and speed differentials. At the slower end of the spectrum you have the saddle-rack that

averages from 6 – 10 mph with a shuffling step behind and a slight lifting (steppy) stride in the front. In this variation of the rack the suspended weight transfer happens with barely any aerial phase. As a matter of fact you may have to look close, and listen closer, to determine if indeed a horse may be racking or fox-trotting or moving in a stepping pace. It is quite common at this slower shuffling saddle rack that a horse may appear very close to the foxtrot with broken diagonal timing, or they can swing the entire spectrum of timing and to carry a laterally timed, broken pace.

Few clinicians seem ready to acknowledge or discuss that there is also this added variation of *TIMING* within the racking gaits that range of from broken pace to broken trot with the majority being on the lateral side of that scale. I have observed that the faster a rack is carried the more laterally paired it tends to become, primarily because the lateral pairing supports a faster, more forward movement while the diagonal pairing supports easier loft and upward lift. It is this wide range of timing that confuses many who want to pigeon-hole the rack into a neat little category.

The rack requires a lot of tension in both hips and shoulders to support the suspended weight transfer. As we pointed out earlier tension and brace is produced from muscles contracting in opposition. If the horse braces more equally with dorsal and ventral muscles it supports a more level posture through his core and his rack tends to be more isochronal in timing. If the ventral muscling is more dominant, giving his core a more rounded carriage it is common to see a fox-rack, which is a rack with more diagonal pairing. When the dorsal muscles dominate the tension (more common with the speedier racking gait) the resulting hollow form will tend to push the timing of his rack toward lateral pairing. Though my comparisons speak of rounding, leveling and hollowing of the core, I still assert it is actually the dominance of muscles that is more responsible for the actual timing variances.

What exactly defines a gait as a rack? The tension in the core, with the very fixed head and neck carriage, along with the key fact that *BOTH FRONT AND BACK SUPPORTING PAIRS OF LEGS TRANSFER THEIR WEIGHT WITH A JOGGING MOMENT OF AERIAL SUSPENSION*, all the while maintaining a four-beat footfall. It is this suspended weight

transfer that creates the signature one-hoof support for each of the hooves in the stride rotation. Never do both hooves of either supporting pair remain in weight bearing contact with the ground at the same time in a rack. Therefore you should never see a three hoof support moment. If you do, you are evidently looking at a different gait.

Please note that many saddle racks can be so low energy and relaxed that they appear to the naked eye to have both hooves in ground contact at once, however if you observe closely you see the telltale signs of suspended weight transfer that indicates they never bear weight at once. If no weight is being born by both hooves there is an aerial phase even if it is brief and difficult to detect.

All racking gaits will exhibit a 2-1-2-1-2-1 hoof support sequence, confirming there is never a 3 hoof supporting moment. There are even rumored to be horses that can actually extend both speed and loft of the racking gait to the point of a ***true single hoof support at all times***. However I've personally never witnessed high definition video evidence to prove there is *NEVER* more than one hoof on the ground at any moment throughout the stride rotation. I'm not saying it can't happen, but I am from Missouri after all, and I'm afraid you're going to have to 'show me'. I will confirm that it is the lofting aerial weight transfer that opens up extreme speed potential for this gait, and that ***the greater the speed the longer the aerial phase will become.*** So, theoretically, the single hoof support throughout the stride rotation is possible.

Much like we can walk at a variety of speeds, there is a definite range most of us will be unable to extend beyond while remaining at the walk. However, once you change your carriage to include a running or leaping step, you have opened up your speed from a 3 mph jog to a 20+ mph sprint. Likewise when a horse transitions into the suspended strides of the rack he opens the door to extreme speed potential.

FEEL FROM THE SADDLE

The rack has a unique and quite addictive feel when ridden. Liz Graves called it the *"eye of the hurricane"* because of the busy sensation both front and back that are in opposite time with each other. I say it's much like sitting in the middle of a teeter-totter where both ends are working in opposition while you sit quietly in the middle. It also has a definite floating sensation due to the complete suspension in both supporting pair of legs during their weight transfers. When a horse morphs or lifts into the rack you feel like someone just switched on a hovercraft beneath you. This floating sensation coupled with the excessive speed potential of this gait makes it a favorite among pleasure riders.

The slower saddle racks are very relaxed and often quite effortless for the horse. Many can build their endurance levels to support this gait for a lengthy go between breaks. The speedier, single-foot racks however require a tremendous amount of energy and should be asked for sparingly on open ground while allowing frequent breaks for your horse to recover. The more rigid topline coupled with an often higher head carriage combines to create a gait that is not as fluid or adaptable to uneven ground, so consequently a racking horse may tend to stumble more often.

I enjoy the rack and will train this gait on each of my finished horses once their skeletal structure is fully mature and they have become set in all their signature gaits. I have yet to find any gaited horse that cannot learn to rack. Indeed, many are so pre-disposed by both breeding and temperament to utilize this gait that once they've become used to it, it can be hard to get them to do anything else. For most pleasure riders this is not a problem and they are quite happy to cruise along riding this pleasurable easy gait.

Part II – PARNTERSHIP OF RIDING

It is important for every rider to give some thought about what kind of relationship they want to have, and how much of themselves they are prepared to invest into their horse. I will admit that horsemanship may not be the best hobby, sport or passion for a totally results oriented personality. You should approach it with a full realization that you are not the only factor or variable. Your horse will be bringing his or her own temperament and personality into the mix, and we, as the trainer/leader should be willing to work with whatever abilities our horse brings as long as those abilities are offered willingly. Training our horses to improve and become more than they now are should be a passionate endeavor where we seek the small successes and embrace any and all effort.

There is a vast difference between working with your horse and making your horse. I believe most of us understand this difference. We may question at times if we're being too soft to achieve results, and begin to consider that maybe we need to be more assertive to get this horse to understand. Well let me reassure you this is rarely the case. A horse that performs to avoid corporal punishment is a much different animal than one who wishes to please and is looking for affirmation and reward. Do not take this to mean that you should be a total cupcake. You still need to be the leader of the relationship and demonstrate a willingness to lead.

While I'm not one to dismiss any trainer's effort *YOU, AS OWNER,* have the opportunity and ability to establish an unmatched connection with your horse over the years that a short term or temporary trainer cannot achieve. It's a partnership that can and should grow stronger with each year you spend together. A trainer simply cannot establish this type of deep bond in the short amount of time most of us will be working with your horse. But like any relationship, your partnership with your horse needs to have an honest foundation

of understanding for both of you to feel comfortable with your roles.

I will frequently refer to the partnership with your horse as your contract with him, for that is in essence what it is. While you should be the leader of the relationship, like any other contract there exists reciprocal responsibilities. *BOTH PARTIES CONTRIBUTE AND BOTH PARTIES BENEFIT.* Once your horse begins to learn and understand the nature of your communication it becomes a game in which most are very willing to participate and partner with you.

Your biggest challenge is to cross that communication barrier between yourself, a predominantly verbal communicator, and your horse, a predominantly non-verbal communicator of body language. As the leader it is up to you to take the initiative for speaking a language your horse can understand: to know what you want, to be clear and consistent in how you communicate it. A common mistake riders make is not being aware of their horse's ability to read your body language. Some riders focus so intently on what they *THINK* they are asking while being completely oblivious to their body language and what it's telegraphing to their horse.

Use trailer loading as an example. You're getting ready to go somewhere and you're anticipating your horse will be difficult about getting into the trailer because he has been in the past or maybe you've never loaded him by yourself before. Furthermore you have a schedule and you don't have a ton of spare time. Naturally you're somewhat tense and anxious about whether or not you're going to be able to get your horse into your trailer easily and in short order. Your horse **reads** this anxiety and thinks *YOU ARE UNCERTAIN ABOUT THE TRAILER AND WORRIED ABOUT GOING IN YOURSELF.* He's not sure but he can tell you're worried and if his person is worried then he better hold up to think about this whole trailer thing. Even if you walk in first he's still aware of your tense posture, your increased respiration, the tension in your face and shoulders, the expression around your eyes. He's still reading fear and worry in these body signals, and figures that if you're afraid of that trailer he should be too. In short, be aware of the unintentional signals of your body language. You must learn to be a mime and aware that working with horses it's always a game of charades.

When I trailer train my young horses I set aside at least 30 minutes for the lesson though it rarely actually takes that long, and I'm able to be totally relaxed about however long it does take because I don't actually have to go anywhere. I arm myself with treats only for reward, never to bribe them into the trailer. I have them on a long line with a rope halter so they are less likely to try to drag me back to the barn if they get too worried. Then I climb into the trailer, lean against the wall and apply very light asking pressure to the line, all the while acting like I'm about to doze off. I slump, yawn, even let my eyes appear drowsy, sigh and just keep asking while waiting patiently *like I have all day*. Sometimes I even take a seat on the floor of the trailer. Anyway, soon my curious little friend is thinking "Huh!" sniffing and looking closely, until he soon decides he's ready to be with me, steps right on up and *THAT's* when he gets the treat. We back out

and repeat a few more times until he thinks it's a game. I bring him back for a refresher a couple of times later that week or the next but he's got it by then and it's no worries. What's the moral of the story? Your body language is an effective communicator with your horse. Be aware of it and use it to your advantage.

You've heard me talk about the contract that we negotiate with our horses. Well it is this contract with your horse that expresses and defines what natural horsemanship is all about. Your agreement to ask him for his cooperative effort and his willingness to comply as long as you keep his best interests at heart.

Don't get frustrated if you have to frequently re-establish ground that you felt has already been covered. If we go for a short while without riding, particularly with the younger, greener horses, we need to give them some refreshing on some of the basics. That's why riding and training is a hobby as well as a passion for most of us. If we wanted absolutes, we'd probably be riding bicycles or driving some kind of mechanical form of transportation. It is the challenge of working within this contract we've established to see just how much we can get our horse to give us.

Chapter 3 – Responsibilities of Partnership

As the leader of the partnership you wish to establish with your horse, you will have the majority of the responsibility as well as the direction. You have three fundamental responsibilities.

HORSE'S COMFORT

By far, our primary responsibility to this partnership is our horse's comfort. This covers everything from the health and soundness of our horse to the equipment we expect him to work with. In a nutshell it is our responsibility

BITTING

Probably the single area that many riders inadvertently create discomfort and stress their horse is in the bit they chose to use. I cannot stress strongly enough how vital it is to use a mild bit that IS COMFORTABLE FOR YOUR HORSE. The bit you choose represents your commitment to communicate and train your horse, and demonstrates how important it is for him to be relaxed and easy with this critical piece equipment. After all y0u're placing hard steel in his mouth and expecting him to carry it with the most delicate tissue on his body.

There are two concerns in bitting a horse that coincide directly with the two major parts of bit construction; the shanks and the mouthpiece. The mouthpiece is what makes

- To make certain your horse is comfortable, physically and mentally
- To know exactly what you want and expect *before you ask*
- To ask for what you want in a consistent manner

to be certain that he is able to fulfill his responsibility without discomfort, pain or stress. He will never fully trust or engage with you emotionally if he is unsure about your commitment to his comfort and well-being.

the most contact and has the most direct influence of how comfortable the bit is for your horse at all times. It is what he wears and carries even when you're not actively making a connection. It should have both the desired fit and action for your horse's comfort and the type of riding you wish to do.

First the bit needs to fit the horse's mouth. This requires a basic understanding of your horse's mouth conformation as well as how a bit sits and is supported within that mouth.

My first advice is to get in there, look and feel. Lift a lip and study how his front upper and lower teeth meet smoothly and should slide easily against each other. These are for biting and tearing up forage. Behind these teeth lay a bare gum gap in front of his back molars called the bars. The bars give us a very handy access to stick our fingers across to measure size and shape of the tongue, how it rests between his jawbones and how high it protrudes above those bars. Also you want to note how highly arched or shallow the palate or roof of his mouth is. Both of these measurements are key, because they tell you what kind of mouthpiece will help your horse be most comfortable. While there is a wide variety of jaw line shapes and sizes within the equine breeds, it is typical that the depth of the tongue rises above the bar line of the lower jaw and if your bit does not allow for this higher arch over the tongue it will rest the bulk of its weight, as well as any pressure you apply directly onto his tongue rather than the sturdier bars of his gums. It is important to know that constriction to the tongue can inhibit his ability to move it and swallow comfortably. There is much debate about at what point bit pressure does inhibit this natural need to swallow, so I'll not get into that here. I will simply say that FOR YOUR HORSE'S COMFORT he should be able to move his tongue and that the majority of the bit weight and pressure should fall onto the bars when the bit is not engaged by the reins. Only by giving him a bit to wear that allows for some freedom to the tongue will you be giving your horse every opportunity to be comfortable. Any bit that is straight across with no lift will rest its weight and any rein pressures on the tongue of your horse. Some bits are actually designed to do just that and work exclusively off of tongue pressure. I find these bits to be unforgiving and will often encourage a horse to get behind the bit and hold his face behind the vertical to avoid that bit contact and pressure.

Tongue relief brings up another area that I've not heard addressed anywhere else as yet. IT IS THE NEED FOR FREEDOM OF THE TONGUE SO THAT A WALKING HORSE CAN NOD HIS HEAD. Huh? Yes, that's right. Your gaited horse, benefits in having freedom for his tongue

to move, improving his ability to nod his head unimpeded at the flatfoot walk. An anatomy study discussed in an article written by Dr. Joyce Harman, DVM, MRCVS titled ***Anatomy and Physiology of the Mouth as it Relates to Bits,*** shows that the tongue is actually a long organ directly attached to a series of small bones at the back of the jaw named the Hyoid bones. There are two major muscles originating at the Hyoid bones that reach back through the front of the neck to the sternum, and another that runs to the shoulder of the horse. This demonstrates a direct connection from the tongue to both the sternum and the shoulder. Dr. Harmon asserts that the relaxation of the tongue exerts direct affect on both the relaxation and the free movement of the shoulder and poll areas.

"All of this anatomy and physiology translates into a horse that is able to move more freely and with better coordination when his tongue is free and soft. Horses' strides can lengthen significantly, their balance becomes better and above all they are softer to ride."

Dr. Joyce Harman, DVM, MRCVS

Ever wonder why some gaited horses will relax into the flatfoot walk and click their teeth? Well my epiphany moment happened as I watched several horses walking in a very relaxed movement and a few were clicking their teeth, while I noticed others were actually licking at the ground with every downward nod of their head. Let me stress these horses were moving very relaxed with total release in their jaws being ridden on loose reins while showing absolutely no resistance. It was quite a sight to see horses walking, nodding and licking, their tongues extending through their lips at the bottom of each nod. Since seeing this in these first couple of horses, I've started noticing it more and more when watching a flatfoot walk from the ground. This awareness started me researching. It was when I realized that the tongue had its direct attachment to the sternum and the shoulder I began to understand that a horse's head movement was applying pull and release on his tongue via these same muscles; and that as long as he is very relaxed in this carriage and not braced against the bit he will feel a natural inclination to move that tongue forward and backward with the headnodding motion. If you have the bit weight resting on his tongue rather than on the bars as it should, this natural movement for both the headnod and the tongue will be restricted or inhibited. Dr. Harman also asserts that tongue discomforts will likely cause stiffness through his shoulders as well as his neckline.

The width of a bit is pretty self explanatory. If too wide, it will wallow causing its action to be distorted and any pressure misapplied. There is also the risk of abrading the corners of the lips if the mouthpiece does not connect smoothly to the shank. If the bit is too narrow its action will be restricted and the lips may become pinched. Width is simple to measure. Tie a string around a pencil, pull the string through to the point where the pencil rests *LIGHTLY* along the side of his mouth and pinch the string with your fingers where it comes free of the opposite side. Remove the string and measure from pencil to your fingers. This will give you *THE MINIMUM* width needed for the mouthpiece and you should try to stay ¼"and no more than 1/2" wider than this measurement.

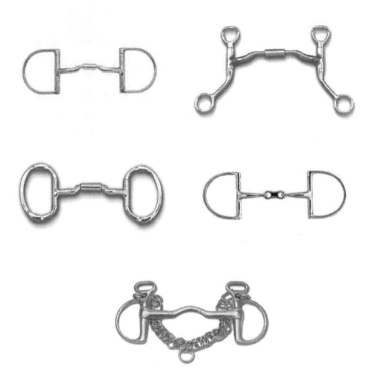

Figure 3.1

In my experience the most comfortable and well accepted mouthpieces for gaited horses are constructed of at least 3 pieces, with a raised center for tongue allowance. Note that some horses prefer the feel that a solid mouthpiece provides. If that is the case with your horse, I recommend trying a low port solid mouth or a mullen mouth that has a natural arch over the tongue. All of these mouthpieces provide consistent tongue relief and place the weight of the bit onto the bars.

Beware that the concept of a port can be

carried too far. I would avoid anything raised more than ¾ of an inch as I have yet to find a gaited horse that has that high an arch to his palate. A low port somewhere around ¼ to ½ inches is usually quite sufficient and comfortable. I recommend trying a number of bits to find what your horse is happiest with if at all possible. I totally understand that this can be somewhat expensive, and recommend either finding a dealer that will let you try it through a loaner program or learn to buy and sell through EBay. A quality bit does not lose its value simply because it doesn't fit your horse and can often be resold for almost the purchase price. Remember that the bit is a long lasting investment and the better made bits even more so. While purchasing a quality bit for your horse may seem to be a splurge, the reality is that once you've found that well fitting bit that your horse is comfortable with, you are set for many years in most cases.

I am *NOT* a fan of any single joint mouthpiece in promoting comfort for the horse. Their action is borderline rude to most horses, and I put single joints in the realm of a correction bit rather than a good communication tool. While many trainers may not concur I will say that the vice-like action is not agreeable to me and its action will naturally apply greater pressure to the more sensitive sides of the tongue rather than the center. The action of the mouthpiece is likely to pinch the most sensitive area of the horse's mouth and these bits will not be considered as part of my partnership agreement with horses that I train.

Also please avoid any bit with the term <u>wire</u> in the name. When it comes to bitting anything extreme will be uncomfortable. Too thin and it becomes cutting and abusive. Too wide and it becomes bulky and does not allow the mouth to rest comfortably closed. My advice is to go with no diameter thinner than ¼ inch and nothing wider than ½ inch in a steel mouthpiece. The rubber mouthpieces can be a little more acceptable at a larger ½ to 5/8 inches, but even those will become difficult for a horse to carry with comfort in any diameter greater than that.

The shanks are the second bit feature for consideration and determine the action that the reins apply to that vital mouthpiece being carried by your horse.

A snaffle bit is any bit that has shanks composed of one ring on each side to which both the reins and head stall are attached. Contrary to the popular misnomer often used by western bit manufacturers to promote the idea that their curb bit is mild by calling it a snaffle, *A TRUE SNAFFLE BIT HAS NO CURB OR LEVERAGED ACTION,* and comes in all varieties of mouthpieces, even the solid mouth low port I recommended above.

Is it a Snaffle bit?

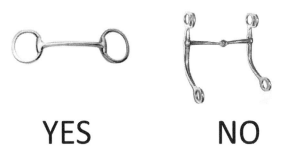

YES   NO

Figure 3.2

Snaffle bits are also called "direct action" bits because they act upon the mouthpiece with pull from "one direction", that of the reins. For this very reason it the optimal bit for training by making the movement you desire clearer and more "direct". I am a firm believer in training with snaffle bits and rarely only progress to a leveraged curb at the point I am beginning to canter a horse. Why confuse your horse with seemingly conflicting pressures? Remember that bits are a communication tool not a brake or steering wheel. A big part of riding in a snaffle is you learning to ride without the corporal force of a curb bit. You will need to educate yourself to disengage the horse through bending when encountering unpredictable obstacles or worrisome actions. Those types of situations will always be encountered and are an undeniable part of riding horses. Making the commitment to train yourself to ride with a snaffle will make you a better rider in the end. Be sensible and start in a controlled, enclosed area and only expand that area as you are assured of your ability to deal with surprise movements and can disengage the horse's backend. Even if you only use the snaffle when in an arena setting both you and your horse will benefit from its use.

Conversely a curb bit acts upon the horse's head in three different directions. When you pull on the rein the mouthpiece presses down onto the tongue and bars, the curb strap or chain pulls up against the jawbone, and the leveraged action of the purchase (that portion of the shank that is above the mouthpiece) pulls downward on the headstall applying pressure on the horse's poll. Some curb bits also employ severe mouthpieces that further action harshly

SADDLE FIT

Nowhere else is more money spent *LESS EFFECTIVELY* than in the purchase of a saddle for a gaited horse. You want to love what it looks like, and you definitely want it to function for your desired discipline or activity, but

on the inside of the horse's mouth. Such is the spade bit that is designed to only allow the horse to be without discomfort if overly flexed when the rider applies contact.

Simply put a curb bit is designed to ask for a finished movement. It is designed to take light, small fingertip movement and translate that into a subtle give at the poll desired in a more finished horse. I advocate training this movement to the horse first with a snaffle bit and teaching your horse rather than forcing him into headset by using more bit than he's ready for.

There are thousands of bit designs out there with more coming out ever year, most of which are marketed to control the horse rather than ask. It is appalling the inhumane tactics employed by people whose only thought is to enjoy their horse and have been told by someone they trust to use this or that bit to get their desired control or action from their horse. Please just get back to the training arena and TRAIN YOUR HORSE. Don't listen to the advice that *"if you have a problem with your horse you just need a bigger bit."* The bit you choose demonstrates exactly how committed you are to maintaining your horse's best interest and well-being over what is expedient and convenient. It will take longer to train your horse while learning yourself, but you need to keep in mind that training is an investment in your relationship and part of your contract. Please read the chapter on bit training for more about this vital part of the relationship with your naturally gaited horse. Make him comfortable and work with his mind and you'll be on the road to developing the partnership you're looking for.

much like a lovely pair of shoes you see in a catalogue, even if you purchase your size they often will be atrociously uncomfortable and will end up sitting in your closet unused. Our horses do not have the luxury of choosing not to wear a poor fitting saddle, and must endure whatever we put on their backs. The saddle we choose for them becomes not only a primary indication of how seriously we accept our responsibility to their well-being and comfort, but the comfort of their back is extremely key to a gaited horse's ability to maintain the relaxed, neutral topline that allows them to gait closer to the desired even four beat that gives us the smooth ride we want.

There are so many dimension to good saddle fit that it is understandable why there is tremendous confusion. To properly fit a horse to a saddle it is essential to understand the movement needed for whatever gait that horse executes. While all horses walk under saddle and execute independent movement of all four quadrants in that more sedate gear, our gaited horses ratchet up their energy level while maintaining similarly independently movement of their quadrants during their faster intermediate gaits. Added to this is the fact that many gaited breeds have inherently longer reach and stride that mandates greater extension of the limbs which directly translates into more roll, twist, torque and overall

movement through the topline. This increased topline movement should be a *SIGNIFICANT CONSIDERATION IN FITTING THEIR SADDLES*.

Unfortunately, far too many of the traditional saddle makers take the same tree they have been manufacturing for decades for their stock saddles and dress them up with shorter, rounded skirting and deeper panels on the front then call it a gaited saddle. Do your homework and learn the basics of saddle fit as well as the movement needed for the way you ride your horse before choosing, and fitting, a saddle. This is your responsibility in the partnership with your horse. He certainly has little say in the matter of what saddle you throw on his back.

I've always been an advocate of *FITTING THE HORSE FIRST*. You can have the highest performance car in the world, but without quality tires all that performance becomes pretty meaningless. Also is the fact that there is much we can do to a saddle to make it more comfortable and convenient for us, but the tree really needs to fit the horse's back or he's just plain miserable and sore and may become unruly or fractious.

IMPORTANT FEATURES OF SADDLE FIT

Please understand that the entire purpose of a saddle is not (contrary to what some people might believe) to give us something to hang a saddle bag on. Its true purpose is to distribute our weight from one concentrated point (our seat bones) and spread it over a greater area along with the associated pressure, while allowing us to maintain a balanced and independent seat. The greater area you can spread weight the easier it generally becomes to support that weight, but there are a few exceptions and concerns.

Some elements of a saddle are of more concern for the comfort of the rider such as depth of seat, cushioning, twist, design, accoutrements, and tooling and I'll let you decide which of those are more suitable for

your riding needs. Some features *ARE MORE VITAL TO YOUR HORSE'S COMFORT*. I'm a firm believer in *FITTING THE HORSE FIRST*. Your horse has no choice in the matter and we should remember it is *our responsibility* to make them as comfortable as we can.

No horse's back is perfectly flat. While relaxed and standing square the highest point of the back of a mature horse is normally the withers. In immature horses the highest point is often at the sacrum. The thoracic vertebrae of the withers have longest spinous processes which are longer and elevate higher above the shoulders. These processes shorten as they slope backward through the last vertebra in the thoracic chain. The thoracic vertebrae are supported by the ribs and their processes are angled backward. The lumbar vertebrae are next in line with no supporting ribs beneath them and with spinous processes that are angled more forward. They rise gradually upward toward the sacrum and have more downward flexion due to both the lack of rib support as well as the shorter spinous processes. The downward and upward sloping lines will normally produce a somewhat smooth curve to the spine that our saddle needs to fit.

LENGTH OF PANELS will greatly affect how large an area the weight of the rider and saddle get distributed to and what region of the back bears that weight. Where many saddle designs go wrong is lengthening the panels to provide greater distribution of the weight, while not considering that the lumbar and the thoracic areas of the back handle that weight differently. The thoracic vertebrae are supported by the rib cage which reinforces them and is a tremendous help in bearing weight. The spinous processes are shorter on the lumbar vertebrae behind the thoracic vertebrae, and therefore they allow more downward flex and drop in that portion of the back. Simply put the lumbar area is more flexible and not as sturdy. A consequence of this flexion is the dorsal muscles must tighten to support any significant weight placed upon this less sturdy region of the back. As discussed earlier, tightening of the dorsal muscles often produce dorsal dominance which promotes lateral gait and pacing in the gaited horses.

Therefore we need to feel for that last rib and follow it upward to where it attaches, then make every attempt to keep the weight of our saddle forward of that point. Too much weight behind the thoracolumbar (T-L) juncture will encourage the horse to drop his back and make the desired neutral topline more difficult.

Cutback saddles, commonly used with gaited horses in saddleseat discipline are specifically designed to place a rider's weight at the very back of the saddle. Added to that structure is the more forward alignment of the stirrups that will further encourage a backward bracing or chair-seat that will focus the rider's weight at the furthest portion of the seat. The design as well as the name *cutback* tend to focus your thinking about freeing the withers and keeping saddle pressure off of them, which is fine by itself. Unfortunately many people do not pay attention to exactly where these saddles ***do place*** their weight. Indeed, many performance horse riders desire this backward weight placement to actually encourage the very action most of us are concerned about. Their desire is to promote a more laterally timed gait. I address this in more detail in the chapter on rehabilitating the performance horse.

Saddles designed for the larger warm blood and dressage breeds inadvertently place weight too far back on our gaited horses with their shorter topline. Pay particular attention to those English saddles that are designed and built with added gussets extending behind the seat, for they will do exactly that. So, too, do many of the western pleasure saddles with large square skirting. Rounded up shorter panels are often a better fit for our gaited horses as well as rounder skirting on the trail and western saddle styles.

ROCK is just as it sounds, the upward curve in the tree panels that should somewhat mimic the curve and contour of the horse's back. The reason I list this first is because it is one of the more hidden elements of fit and, as such, one of the most frequently overlooked.

Looking at the bareback topline of this horse in the top-most photo you can see a natural curvature behind the withers that is created by the spinous processes of the spine. In many gaited breeds this curvature is even more dramatic than we see here with this young walking horse. This curved alignment becomes an important feature to consider in saddle fit.

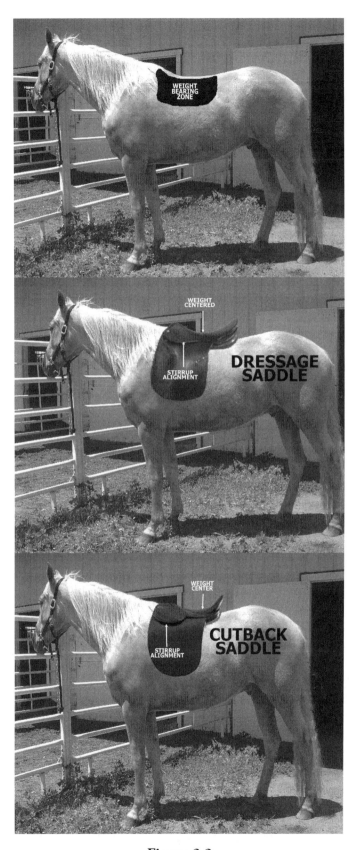

Figure 3.3

If the saddle has more curve than a horse's topline, rather than diffuse the weight of the rider it will instead concentrate the weight of both rider and saddle onto a too small area which does little to spread the weight and reduce the pressure. Too much rock can focus the weight and become painful to a horse over many miles and hours. However, if the saddle has less curve (is flatter) than the back of the horse it may cause bridging where the weight of the rider and saddle get distributed outward away from the center to the front and back of the saddle and creates a bridge over the most solid portion of the back. I believe bridging is more common in our gaited horses because many have prominent withers and tend to be conformed with a significant curve through their thoracic vertebrae. Bridging focuses the weight of rider and saddle toward the extreme points of contact at both the shoulders and the unsupported lumbar vertebrae of the back, while bridging across the center with little or no weight there where we actually want the primary weight bearing area to be. Many trees are designed for non-gaited horses that will have more lift through their core to encourage rounding for the trot, and if you are riding a trotting horse it is worth considering. Many gaited horses travel with level or even slightly hollow thoracic vertebrae that cannot support the needed weight when the saddle is bridging. While we want to encourage our gaited horses to lift their midline to occasional light rounding most of our isochronal gaits will be carried with a neutral or natural posture for his conformation and a saddle that fits that conformation is needed to accommodate this with even pressure. Topline fit, or rock, is a critical problem without a simple answer because gaited horses come in a variety of sizes and conformations that make the entire one-tree-to-fit-all-gaited-horses a myth. Neither too much nor too little rock is acceptable for the fit of your horse because his comfort directly affects how he carries his back and consequently the gait he's giving you. If your saddle maker, or saddle fit advisor does not take the rock of the saddle and the curve of the horse's topline under primary consideration, it could very well be detrimental to the gait he's able to give you.

FLARE is a widening of the saddle tree panels as they progress forward (back to front) toward the withers or pummel. The panels need to be aligned flatter toward the rear of the saddle and more vertical as well as more open (apart) toward the front to accommodate the increased slope near the withers and allow the shoulders to rotate uninhibited. You should be able to follow the shoulder scapula from its lower point upward where it crowns near the wither while the saddle is in place. In many horses this scapula (equivalent to the human shoulder blade) will be as large as a spread hand near its crown. Feel and find this scapula and note its placement. Then understand that this bone needs to rotate as a horse moves and will need another inch all around the perimeter for clearance. When your saddle is placed and cinched it will need to flare out away from this boney structure and you should be able to snuggle your fingers over and around it *WITH THE SADDLE CINCHED INTO PLACE*. If you cannot then your saddle does not have enough flare to allow freedom for your horse's shoulder. Pinching against the scapula will inhibit a horse from rolling well and reaching forward with his frontend as well as generally being uncomfortable in his saddle.

Another consideration of **flare** is the angle of the front of the panels and many people only consider this feature and not the actual clearance of the scapula. In a perfect world the angle of the saddle panels should match the slope of the shoulder alignment creating a larger area of contact. As we mentioned above the greater the contact area the less pressure will be applied to any one point.

One common mistake is sliding the saddle back away from the shoulder to where the saddle settles. While this may free up the scapula, it places the saddle in a position where the rest of the contact becomes a very poor fit and will create more problems than it solves. It also places almost all saddles too far back onto the unsupported lumbar vertebrae which are weaker and often drop under pressure which forces the dorsal muscles to contract to increase support. As discussed previously, braced dorsal muscles will invariable lead to a pacing problem at gait.

A very common error in thinking about saddle fit is to pad up a tight fitting shoulder to cushion and protect the horse from saddle pressure. *The Cardinal Rule of Saddle fit:* **additional padding or thickness increases pressure while reduction of thickness or padding reduces pressure.** It is so important to understand that wherever the saddle fit is too tight or is making too much contact the last thing you should do is add more padding to this pressure point. Added padding simply exacerbates the fit problem by placing more bulk where the fit is already too tight. You should only add padding where the saddle makes little or no contact to increase pressure and share the load. This process is called shimming. Successful shimming requires padding up areas to increase pressure and relieve other areas that are over burdened. It is common to shim beneath the rider when a saddle bridges. This will often slightly lift the rest of the saddle off those areas being over burdened and actually lighten the shoulder fit and weight being placed there as it increases the contact and weight burden to the area being shimmed.

Gullet width and depth is what accommodates the spine of the horse in the area forward of the rider's seat. The panels of a saddle need to flare apart and lift upward so they do not interfere with the needed movement of either the withers or the shoulders. Most saddle trees are labeled and identified by the width of this gullet measurement in stated centimeters, inches, narrow, medium, wide or extra-wide.

Gaited horses often have prominent withers and many mistakenly believe that the high bony ridge indicates the need for a high, narrow gullet. While it does indicate that your horse requires a deep gullet and saddles with a little more rock to the panels will likely fit best, *THE TRUE WIDTH NEEDED IN THE GULLET IS FOR THE SHOULDER MEASUREMENT BELOW THE WITHERS.* The scapula is the upper bone of the front leg and runs from the point of the shoulder to align *near* the crown of the withers. Notice I say near because the shoulder does not actually connect to the spine through any boney joint, only through muscles and ligaments. It is this separation that allows the scapula to move more freely, as well as allowing the energy of the hindquarters to flow uninhibited along the spine through to the headnod. If you can stand in front of your horse and see the increased width at the top of the scapulas you will understand why a wide or extra wide saddle tree is often the best fit for many of these horses. Far too many are being forced to work in saddles that do not allow their shoulders to move freely.

Another thing to consider is if the saddle is too wide it will settle lower and interfere with the wither cap and the support angle near the scapula will be off. If the gullet is too narrow it will pinch the scapula and your horse will find it uncomfortable to roll loosely and reach well with his front legs. The weight of the saddle or rider should <u>never</u> rest or impinge upon either the rotating scapula we call the shoulder or the boney ridge of the spine at the withers.

Spine clearance is so very critical to your horse's comfort, and again it is often unnoticed or completely disregarded. The channel between the panels of a saddle is what allows the vertebrae to move freely without bearing any weight. Historical thinking has been that three fingers width between the panels are adequate for this movement, but more recent research is indicating that the need for bend through the spine requires the clearance should actually be greater and now recommends four fingers width.

DEPTH OF THE CHANNEL is also of critical concern for those horses' that have a more prominent profile to their spine. Whether this is due to conformationally longer spinous processes of the vertebrae or atrophied muscling along either side of the spine or possibly even body condition being below optimal makes little difference. The solution is the same: to build up the areas on either side and increase the pressure onto the ribs while reducing any possible pressure to the spine. There are exercises to help the muscling somewhat, but your first responsibility is to *MAKE CERTAIN YOUR HORSE'S SPINE IS NOT SUPPORTING ANY DIRECT WEIGHT OF THE SADDLE OR RIDER.* I highly recommend utilizing cutout saddle pads that have a relief channel formed down the midline to provide freedom of movement for the spine.

If you are uncertain how much clearance your current saddle provides to your horse I recommend aligning a typical lead rope along the spine, under your saddle. When your saddle is cinched down, you should still be able to easily pull the lead rope out. If you cannot do this then you need to be concerned that your horse is experiencing pressure directly on the vertebrae of his spine. This pressure may completely lock him up as he resists any movement that will aggravate the vertebrae.

GIRTH RIGGING is more than just a way to secure your saddle. It's a huge variable, limited somewhat by saddle design that is very crucial to how the saddle is positioned, balanced and carried by the horse. A very determined rider can often find solutions to rigging difficulties with a little creativity.

I personally never recommend the single forward full rigging seen on many western saddles. These saddles often aren't a quality fit for your gaited horse anyway, having been constructed with Quarter horse bars. But my personal preference is to balance your saddle as best you can from front-to-back. This is usually accomplished by some variation of a center-fire rigging which more and more of the gaited saddles are being produced with. Center-fire rigging places the girth further away from the front legs which also help in preventing girth gall. But mostly it balances the saddle by connecting to both front and back rigging D's.

If you have a saddle that fits your horse wonderfully but has the full forward rigging I recommend you consider trying a pack cinch that you can rig through both the front and back D's of the saddle. There is not a huge selection of pack cinches available, but more are being produced all the time.

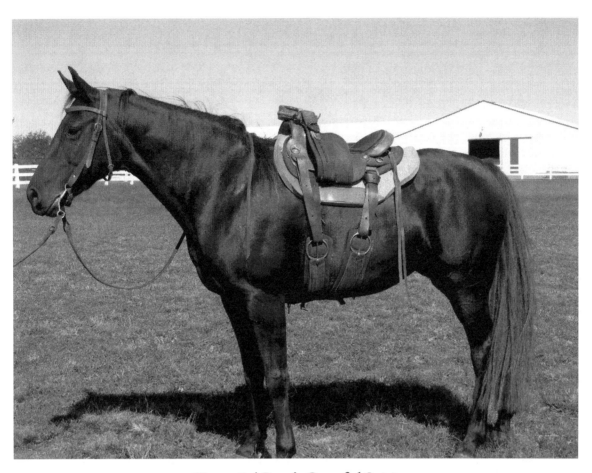

Figure 3.4 Papa's Graceful Spirit

The pack cinch, sometimes called a sawbuck cinch is a double cinch that rigs to both front and back D's on either side of the horse and was originally designed for use with packs that require stabilizing. I do advise one word of caution. If you have never before placed a center-fire rigging on your horse, take care the first time you cinch him up that you allow him to move out freely in a paddock or round pen for a few minutes. There are a few horses that are sensitive enough to the girth being placed a little further back on their belly line who react to that pressure with a few bucks or broncs initially. Make certain that even with the dual pack cinch or whichever center-fire rigging you may chose, *YOU KEEP THE VERY BACK PORTION OF THE GIRTH POSITIONED <u>WELL IN FRONT OF THE HORSE'S UMBILICAL MIDLINE</u>*. Any pressure behind this point may likely trigger a

somewhat violent reaction, and act much like a bucking strap. While a few horses can be sensitive to the wider area of the double girth or the more posterior positioning of any center-fire rigging, most are very tolerant or take no notice of the differences and eventually even prefer this positioning. I use a double pack cinch with all my western saddles and have ridden dozens upon dozens of horses this way and have only come across two that absolutely would not tolerate it.

Another benefit of the double rigging of the pack cinch is that it provides a much greater area of contact with the horse and thereby allows us to be less severe in cinching up the horse. Both of these facts *ADD TO THE COMFORT OF THE HORSE*, which you will recall is our responsibility in the partnership. I have a pack cinch made of soft neoprene that I tighten only enough to maintain secure and firm contact with the horse. This may indeed be a primary reason why, in my experience, most horses learn to prefer these cinches. After all, we are asking them to be athletes and work for us, and I find it completely inhumane to cinch them up so hard that we cut off their ability to breathe deeply and move comfortably. I never want any cinch or girth to be so tight that I cannot pull it away from the horse's

How do I fit my horse?

Like purchasing a quality pair of athletic shoes for aerobics, jogging or any other sport, a poor fit will render even the most expensive pair of shoes pretty worthless. Likewise, a little forethought into fitting our saddles will pay off exponentially.

There are about as many theories on saddle fit as there are saddle makers out there. Many will endlessly blog on their websites about this myth or that vital feature. I do not subscribe to any one saddle maker exclusively, but have found that the features I've discussed here always seem to help my horses be more comfortable and move more freely and some knowledgeable saddle makers understand these needs better than others. When you're asking your horse to carry himself with a relaxed neutral topline it is vital that we do not sabotage his efforts by outfitting him in a miserably uncomfortable saddle.

First take a long and careful look at how your horse is built. Pay attention to both the depth and height of his spine and withers. Look at how round his barrel is and exactly how long his topline is to the thoracic and lumbar vertebral juncture. Take coat-hanger wire and bend it across the top of the withers reaching down over the scapula on each side. Remove and measure the width 11-13 inches down from the peak where those shoulders are located. Study the angle of alignment. Both of these measurements will help you fit the flare

side with a moderate pull; far enough to run my hand beneath it easily. Keep in mind that with many of us who are not light weights, once we mount up the girth will drop looser especially if you have thick padding beneath your saddle. If I have a thick pad I always take a moment to snug up the cinch from on board the saddle. I always recommend using saddle pads but consider it important to check girth contact after you've mounted.

and width of the tree.

The best tool I've found to analyze fit of the saddle rock is an impression pad. This is a clear vinyl saddle pad filled with a soft dough-like substance that will form and maintain an impression when placed under a saddle and ridden for a few minutes. It will completely map the exact fit of any saddle to any horse, and highlight any pressure points by those areas where the dough filling is pushed away showing clear through the vinyl. Some saddle makers and trainers have these to assist their customers with this critical issue of saddle fit. Some venders actually have loaner programs where you can rent the use of the impression pads for a short time.

Please note that if you fit your horse when he is young and immature, or if for any reason your horse changes his size or shape, you will need to periodically recheck your saddle fit. Also please consider that some saddle trees may warp with age and what you thought was a great buy on EBay may turn out to be a complete mistake for your horse.

For further information on saddle fit I highly recommend you invest in a wonderful and well illustrated book by Dr. Joyce Harman, DVM, MRCVS titled ***The Horse's Pain-Free Back and Saddle Fit Book***

My only comment about saddle features relevant to the rider is regarding stirrup and fender placement for a balanced seat.

Be conscious that your saddle places you in an upright balanced posture and keep your legs in a central, equitation positioning. This feature will help you maintain an independent seat and avoid interfering with your horse's balance or inadvertently putting pressure in

SHOEING

Shoeing is the one area where you will find the greatest diversity of opinion when it comes to gait, gaited horses and gait correction. Over decades of horse shows and performance training the idea of enhancing gait with the use of mechanical shoeing practices has not just taken hold, but become the central thinking for any kind of gait modification in both pleasure and performance horses. It is only in recent years that the overwhelming popularity of the pleasure gaited horse has offered an opportunity for those of us who utilize classical training methods for gait correction over this well established belief in mechanical intervention.

So let me make this exceedingly clear and concise as I can. *A horse's hooves should have a naturally balanced trim with any shoes being added for <u>the protection of the hoof only</u>, never for altering or enhancing gait.* Let's not complicate this any more than we need to. If a trainer advises you to add weight, lower or raise the hoof angle or grow more toe, run away! They are not who you want to be listening to. They're not going to help your horse achieve self carriage, they're only offering a quick fix that may very well degrade your horse's orthopedic health over the long run, while demonstrating their lack of knowledge on how to actually train your horse to correct or improve his gait.

Nothing about gait happens only in the feet. Gait happens in the shoulders hips and

AGE

I cannot emphasize how huge a disservice we do our gaited horses by starting them

his mouth in an effort to balance yourself. To be a confident rider you need to learn to be a balanced rider. Anyone who is unsteady in the saddle will find it difficult to become a relaxed and confident rider who is unafraid of releasing your horse into gait.

topline within a horse's support structure. So do yourself and your horse a huge favor and give him a sound hoof appropriate for his size. For most gaited breeds this will mean a front toe length averaging between 3 $^{1/4}$ - 4 inches in length. If you have a 17 ½ hand horse that has a nicely round hoof with 4 ½ inch toes, then that's absolutely fine for him. But if you have a 15 hand horse that has an oval hoof with 4 ½ inch toes then it's time to honestly ask yourself "Why?" If you feel reluctant to trim a 3 ½ inch hoof on a 15 hand horse and it's for anything other than you feel he will be uncomfortable with a short hoof, then you might want to re-assess your own thinking.

I could write pages instructing you on how to mechanically tweak your horse's timing through creative shoeing and trimming, and many trainers do just that. Believe it or not there are reasons why manipulating your horse's timing through shoe weight, hoof angle and break-over have some limited success. However I would not be doing you or your horse any favors by taking you down that road. We must accept the responsibility to train our horse for his benefit as well as our own. It is his responsibility to learn to carry the gait that's been bred into him, and your responsibility to get out of his way and let him. A big part of getting out of his way is giving him a sound sensible hoof, with a natural break-over to work with.

under saddle at young ages; and am truly horrified when I hear of 15 month old yearlings being ridden under saddle. Those who ride babies are severely handicapping the horse's opportunity to be healthy and successful. Yes, some will manage to be OK. But a tremendous percentage of these horses that have been bred for bigger and looser stride are being started younger and younger and unintentionally lamed for life. There are those that treat these animals as disposable and do not blink an eye at pushing them beyond what they can bear. Part of our responsibilities to these horses are to make certain they are mature enough, healthy enough and just plain strong enough to do the jobs we ask of them.

Most two year olds can *PROBABLY* be strong enough to go around a groomed arena with the *AVERAGE SIZED* adult rider at a walk without too many problems… most of them, maybe. But when you place your horse in this situation you're rolling the dice that he will not take a serious stumble; that his balance is good enough to learn to step into lateral turns; or that he will not hit a rough patch in the arena that will cause him to stumble awkwardly. That's all it takes for the soft joints of young horses to pull or strain. Often times those strains heal by adding scar tissue which does not have near the natural elasticity of the healthy original joint tissues. Range of motion is often compromised on this horse for the remainder of his life, and any potential he/she may have had to be shown is completely down the tubes. I commonly see walking horses in particular, of all ages that exhibit a shorter stride on one back leg or the other. We call these "**three legged horses**", and the sad part is that many of them are nicely moving horses otherwise.

Many believe it's a simple matter of conditioning. Wrong! Bone growth happens in layers called growth plates that are situated at the ends of each and every bone in a young horse. These plates create new bone growth by first building cartilage extension at the bone ends within the joints. This cartilage later calcifies into solid bone as new cartilage is produced on top of it. Here's the kicker… *DURING TIMES OF RAPID GROWTH SPURTS THE NEW CARTILAGE GROWTH OUT STRIPS THE RATE OF CALCIFICATION SO THAT THE JOINTS BECOME SOFTER, LESS STABLE AND MUCH MORE SUSCEPTIBLE TO STRAIN AND INJURY.* The risk is highest during times of rapid growth, which naturally coincide with times of plenty in the horse's food source. In other words during the spring and early summer months when the grass is growing strong and lush in many areas of the country these young horses are experiencing their most rapid growth spurts. You can get a pretty good idea when this rapid growth occurs because it is also reflected in the accelerated hoof growth.

Other factors may also affect growth rates. It's common for horses that change habitat will experience rapid and dramatically increased growth if his nutritional intake increases with the new environment. I have had several horses coming to my farm from an environment of scarcity show rapid and dramatic growth in those first several months. If a young horse is suddenly getting more quality nutrition than he's had previously then he's likely to be going through a growth spurt if he's under 6 ½ - 7 years old.

It's not simply a matter of saying growth stops at a certain age, because these bones (growth plates) mature at different schedules. The first general rule is the closer to the ground, the earlier they mature and cease to grow. This is why measuring the length of the cannon bone is an often used method of estimating the mature height on a young horse. That cannon bone stops growing by the time most young horses are 6-8 months of age. This then means that those delicate bones and joints in the spine and hips *ARE THE LAST TO MATURE SOMEWHERE AFTER OR AROUND THEIR 6TH YEAR.* This schedule is further complicated by the anticipated size of the horse. The second general rule is the larger the horse will be, the later in life he will mature and his bones stop growing. So that a 14.3 hand horse might very well have a mature spine at 6 years, while the 17 hand horse may not have a mature spine until 7 to 7 ½ years old.

Please be aware of the need for solid joints and strong backs in order for our gaited horses to be able to move in balanced self-carriage and easily find a neutral topline that allows them to easily carry their four-beat gait. I, personally, start ground work with my youngsters when they turn three years old. I may put a saddle on during the WINTER MONTHS before they turn four years old and start climbing in and out of the saddle, starting, stopping, moving off my legs and bit training. All of this is still in the round pen or a groomed arena setting. Only after I feel the horse is carrying me in balance and responding softly and readily to all of the above will we move from the round pen to the groomed arena. At this point (at or very near 4 years old) I begin working the flatfoot walk. I will work this walking speed, transitioning from trail walk to flatfoot walk and back again, for the next 6 months. It is ONLY when the horse can demonstrate to me that they are solid enough working this speed that I will begin asking for more energy and impulsion; always transitioning up and down to reinforce the importance of rating his speed to my direction. If everything progresses well, I begin working to ask for canter by their 5 yr old winter. *PLEASE NOTE THAT I ASK FOR THE BIGGEST ADVANCES WITH YOUNG HORSES DURING THE WINTER MONTHS WHEN THEY ARE LESS LIKELY TO BE EXPERIENCING GROWTH SPURTS.*

TEETH

I want to point out that good dental care is not just essential for mature horses. I recommend a good dental exam before you first place a bit a young horse's mouth. I further recommend wolf teeth be extracted and a bit seat to be floated onto the front molars before serious bit training is started. For those not familiar, a bit seat is the process of rounding the front corners of the first molars both top and bottom. This creates a smooth groove for the bit to settle into when you make a connection to the bit through the reins.

I require any horse coming to my barn for training to have had a performance dental float within the last 6 months to reduce the risk of having to interrupt his training to address problems with mouth comfort. A problem with the teeth will invariably influence how the horse responds to the bit and how he carries the bit as well as his head while the bit is in his mouth. An inclination to slant his head to one side is a good indicator that he's experiencing discomfort and is unwilling to engage the bit squarely. When this happens you lose part of your connection and communication to this horse. It should be addressed and resolved as quickly as possible. Any inclination to carry the front of his body to one side or the other should cause us to look at the mouth or the bit first.

GENERAL HEALTH

Overall our horses need to be in good flesh, with solid backs and joints and healthy sound hooves when we put them to work. This is the rider's responsibility to understand and evaluate. Remember this is a partnership and while the horse has no idea what's in store for him… we do. Own up and take care of business by taking care of your horse first.

As a trainer I find a health problem is the likely culprit when a horse is brought to me with a particularly disturbing issue such as rearing or bucking. Often the owner has not paid attention to the milder clues the horse has provided and he has had to escalate his objections to the point of becoming dangerous. Be aware and try to anticipate as much as you can.

Underweight horses will not tolerate the tensions of training as well, nor are they as strong for carrying the burden of rider and tack. I have refused to accept horses in training until their body condition has improved.

KNOW WHAT YOU WANT

Right now you are helping to fulfill this responsibility. You are educating yourself on what you should be seeing and expecting from your horse. Though he can read your body language your horse cannot read your mind. He has no idea what you're going to be asking for until you teach him. As the leader of this partnership it is *YOUR RESPONSIBILITY TO KNOW AND UNDERSTAND THE GOALS OF YOUR TRAINING.* You cannot teach what you do not know or understand, at least not with any consistent success.

BE CONSISTENT

There are two areas that frequently trip up amateur riders who do not practically live with their horses the way some of us seem to do. Utilizing a method of communicating gives our horses a primer they can learn to follow. Method gives your horse fundamentals of communication he can rely upon when trying to figure out what you might be asking when you introduce something new. Many natural horsemanship gurus tailor a method and package it for marketing. Why? Because it works and establishes a language between horse and rider.

My riding and training method is to use my seat and legs as much as possible for all requests relating to everything a horse does with his feet while saving the reins and hands for positioning the horse's head and neck, or for capturing forward energy. I utilize a very common Three Leg Positions cue system,

Poor vaccination and deworming schedules along with poor quality feed puts horses at a tremendous disadvantage in being able to focus on the training. Just like a child that is undernourished has trouble doing well in school, so too do horses that are underfed, or unhealthy have difficulty in learning and making the most of your training efforts.

It is also your responsibility to know exactly what movements you're asking for each and *EVERY* time you apply any pressures or cues to your horse, before you apply that pressure. It is vital that you never ask your horse for anything without a complete and specific understanding of what you want him to do. How else will you know exactly when he gives it to you, and know when to release your cue? Again, he's not a mind reader just a body reader.

with a forward position near the girth line; a central position directly below your seat in equitation posture and finally a back position nearer the flank area. I go into much greater detail about this in the chapter on ***Adding the Power Steering***.

It is one thing to tell people to consistently ask for the same movement the same way. It is another for them to understand how to consistently ask for *similar movement* or actions using *similar cues*. The best way to be consistent is to learn and practice a method for communicating with your horse and stay true to that method as best you can. When you need to figure out how to ask for something new, this method will provide you with a basis on how best to ask for this new movement.

It is through the use of a consistent method of riding and asking that we TRAIN OURSELVES to communicate in a consistent manner. This consistency enables our horse to learn our language, and only through this language can we begin to have dialogue with our horse to establish the terms of our partnership.

The second area many slip up on is by failing to remember that we're working with creatures that use body language and reads our movement, posture and actions much closer than we are aware of.

Chapter 4 - Horse's Partnership Responsibilities

Comparatively, the horse's responsibilities to the partnership are much simpler and basic. It is up to us to establish and train him to his responsibilities in our partnership, and like a good boss or parent, not let him get away with poor behavior without correction.

Training horses is very much like raising children. A horse, like a child, will always test their boundaries. They will push the envelope a little and if they get away with that, they'll push it a little further the next time. Just like correcting your child, you do not have to resort to corporal punishment for correction of your horse. Remember the horse's need to be with us and to be comfortable, so we should use those needs to establish our dominance in a non-painful manner. From this position of dominance we can then be as benevolent as we want, as long as we maintain the contract, and make certain he does as well.

Just as a child will love and respect the parent who establishes and maintains the boundaries, so too will our horses likewise love and respect us. But even more than that, if your horse is not convinced of both your authority and your ability to maintain that authority, he will not feel like you can care for him and, more importantly, protect him. This becomes particularly critical when you begin riding him out onto unknown trails or anywhere he sees as a risky situation. When your horse is completely convinced that you are not just the alpha but a strong alpha, he

will feel more confident and secure when you ask him to approach a new obstacle. He will be more certain that you will protect him and that you will always keep his welfare as top priority.

The horse's responsibilities are fewer, but very specific:

- Pay Attention
- Keep doing what he's doing
- Aggression is never allowed

HIS PRIMARY RESPONSIBILITY IS TO ALWAYS PAY ATTENTION TO YOU. You cannot direct a horse whose always staring off into the distance worried about everything else going on around him. I love Dr. Deb Bennett's frequently used analogy where she calls the horse's attention is his "little birdie". She talks about how you want to keep his little birdie sitting on his shoulder right with you, rather than flying off toward other points of interest or concern. We can help our horse keep his attention on us during moments of stress or distraction by asking him to do something simple when we feel his attention begin slipping away. I often will ask him to reposition his head, usually to lower it, whenever I feel he may be getting ready to worry or react to a situation in an undesirable way. Lowering his head not only gives him something else to focus on but helps keep his attention on me. A lower head position also helps him relax and think rather than worry

64

and react.

A thinking horse rather than a reacting horse is our goal. We always want to keep our horses thinking, but the Good Lord made them creatures of reaction during moments of stress. A horse's eyesight allows him to see best in front of him and into the distance when his head is raised, his nose is lifted up. This position allows his eyes to focus along his nose. So when something surprises or concerns him it is COMPLETELY NORMAL and to be expected for him to throw his head up. This is his fright and flight posture where he is most ready to react quickly and instinctively. THE HIGHER A HORSE'S HEAD THE CLOSER HE IS TO HIS REACTIVE NATURE; WHILE THE LOWER HIS HEAD THE MORE THINKING HE IS AND CLOSER TO HIS LOGICAL NATURE. A high head is his worry posture. So when we ask and help him lower his head it not only relaxes and calms him, but helps him connect more to the thinking, logical side of his brain.

Teaching a drop the head cue is one of the first things I do for every horse I work with. It gives me a tool to help that horse move away from his panic button. A high headed horse has his hand over the panic button and is prepared to react quickly with little warning. Let's face it, when true danger is near the horse who reacts without thinking is the one most likely to survive that danger, so it's no wonder these creatures have evolved over the millennia to react now and think later. In the wild the horse that stops to think about a threat is often the one that gets eaten by the predator. But when we are training it is import for us to have a horse that not only focuses and thinks about what we're asking, but is less likely to spook and startle during lesson times as well as on the trail. So we ask him to drop his head, focus on little exercises and move his hand away from his panic button.

The second responsibility for your horse is that **HE SHOULD ALWAYS KEEP DOING WHAT HE'S DOING UNTIL YOU TELL HIM DIFFERENTLY.** If you ask him to stand still, he should remain still until you ask him to move. If you ask him to walk forward, he should continue doing so *at that speed* until you ask for a change. If you ask him to lower his head, he should keep it lower until you ask for something different. It is one of the simplest rules, but also one of the most challenging for the horse to learn. His own nature wants to insert itself into the picture and this is one rule that gets very rusty when a horse goes for a long period without riding or training. During those periods of layoff his nature is to become more self directing as you would expect, and he may need some reminding when you get on again. Patience, persistence and consistent communication will help you maintain this rule.

FINALLY, NO AGGRESSION WILL BE TOLERATED. I define aggression as *any deliberate movement or intention to harm*. Kicking, biting, slamming into you, and whacking you with his head (though sometimes this can be accidental) or any deliberate attempt t0 strike or step on you. Under saddle behavior can also fall into this category such as bucking. Note that rearing up or bolting under saddle are normally NOT aggressive actions. More often they are acts of self preservation and a reaction to fright or pain. Aggression is an act of dominance that is deliberately directed toward you.

You can never ignore this rule or let your horse get by with breaking it. Be honest with yourself. If you realize that you're a cupcake when it comes to discipline, PLEASE go get yourself a trained horse. For both his sake and yours, a horse that is never taught to respect humans as his caretakers and alpha leaders will have a harsh life ahead of him. Such a horse will always need correcting for misbehavior until such time as someone takes him in hand and teaches him otherwise. Any horse who understands their contract with the humans in their life will have a more successful and happy existence with those humans. So you mustn't think of it as disciplining your horse only for your convenience, it's actually more for his well being over the span of his life, and as critical to him as when teaching young children to never play with fire. You should be honest if you are not able or willing to do this and hire a professional to show you how to consistently work with your horse to establish ground rules of behavior. Every horse has to learn to respect the alpha role of the humans in his life.

Chapter 5 –Give is based on Release

A horse will willingly give us what we ask for if we do so within the bonds of a partnership where he has total confidence that if he gives to us he will be rewarded with release.

This applies to everything we do with our horses. If we're asking a horse to move, accept, stop, or yield we must keep in mind the reciprocal nature of our partnership agreement and what we are offering him in return for his compliant and willing effort. The biggest portion of his reward is our RELEASE. These wonderful animals are so often very willing to work with us because for that effort we give them release from whatever cue we apply, and an occasional stroke along his neck. Once we have established ourselves as the alpha partner and reassured him that his well being is a priority with us he gives.

Have you noticed how the alpha horse in a herd is rarely by himself? The rest of the horses naturally follow the alpha for both comfort and protection because that horse has established himself as the leader. If we do the same we can benefit from our horse's willingness and desire to stay with us. As long as we remember to work with him through release we will continue to have his willing partnership. Without this important and willing effort from the horse, every request has the potential to turn into a battle to be won or lost which can be frustrating for both parties,

and counterproductive in allowing the horse to relax and be happy in his work.

None of this is new or revolutionary. It is the same sensible horsemanship as promoted by those I consider the modern fathers of natural training, Tom and Bill Dorrance and Ray Hunt. It is the same classical training that has been successfully used to work with horses for millennia. The actual birth of natural horsemanship stretches back to Xenophon of Athens around 4th century BC, often referred to the original horse whisperer in advocating sympathetic horsemanship. It has been long believed that training should be a partnership of working *with* your horse. Many interpret horsemanship to be the ability to get willing effort from their horse, and consider it a hobby, but many of us consider it a passion and a way of life.

We must first establish the foundation of our agreements with our horse on the ground before seeking to place a saddle on his back. That is the purpose of ground work; to establish the rules of our partnership, and help the horse understand we wish to work in unity with him. Once you have that understanding in the contract, you can progress to teaching the horse the language of the partnership such as move away from pressure or stand still unless I ask you to move which are both elements of yielding.

Teaching Give by using what I call *the Four*

R's of Horsemanship will allow us to establish a contract with the horse that enables him to feel comfortable, which is all any horse wants. Sam Powell once said that ***"a horse (like most prey animals) has three basic needs: comfort, sustenance and sex. The*** STRONGEST ***of these needs is comfort; he will forego both of the others if he feels uncomfortable or threatened".*** So right there we have the key to negotiating our contract with our horse. It is important you understand that I never advocate using discomfort in the form of corporal punishment. I advocate using his natural need to be relaxed and comfortable by ground driving when he wants to be a bully or resistant and when you make him move when and where you direct you establish dominance over his movement that psychologically affirms your natural dominance over the horse. Do not let him rest until YOU say so and only change directions when YOU say so. You can show your horse that you control his feet in this manner. Ground work can be a dominance exercise that establishes you as the alpha leader, and does so with no actual physical contact even though the horse may think you're going to have him for dinner at first. From this position of dominance and strength you can then establish your benevolence through reward, rest, stroking and just standing quietly with him behind your shoulder. This benevolence demonstrates your desire to unify in partnership, and allows him to comfortably hook up with you. You've earned his respect and he should be willing to work with you once you've established this hook up. You can now demonstrate your commitment to always consider his wellbeing first. This is your fundamental contract that you will develop and constantly add to it as your relationship progresses.

Chapter 6 - Four R's of Natural Training

One of my dearest mentors, Bruce Almeida, taught me about training through what he labeled the three R's: Request, Response and Release. I have utilized this for many years and since added a fourth R, Repetition. Within this structure of THE FOUR R's you have a road map to natural training. No matter the labels used, this is the fundamental process by which all natural training occurs with horses. Even equestrian trick training utilizes these same principles when you get down to it.

Before beginning with the four R's of training it's your responsibility to know what you want, make your horse comfortable in doing it, and be vigilantly watchful for any and all honest effort by your horse to give you the action or movement you are seeking.

REQUEST is where you *ask* your horse for a particular action by applying pressure as a cue. While your horse will often read your body language, he cannot really read your mind. So give some thought about how you want to proceed with your request. If the movement you're wanting has something to do with moving his feet, I recommend using pressure somewhere on his body and using your legs from the saddle. If it has to do with where or how he is carrying his head, then quite naturally you would use the reins and bit from the saddle. However you choose to ask, be consistent and patient. Be ready and watchful for his reciprocal effort to respond.

RESPONSE is whatever the horse does after we request, whether right or wrong. Many people believe a horse learns when he responds, but this is NOT the case. His response is his attempt to ask us if this is what we want. *"IS THIS CORRECT?"* Or it may be a fear reaction if we've asked for too much. Please understand your horse may give you many wrong answers before he gives you a more correct response, and you must *BE PATIENT.* Response is *any* attempt made by your horse to give you some kind of answer, right or wrong. What is important is that *WE KEEP ASKING UNTIL HE GIVES US THE CORRECT RESPONSE.* This is also why it's important to give a cue that is not too complex or uncomfortable to maintain, because we must keep up the pressure until he gives at least an attempt toward the correct movement.

For instance, I will ask a horse to step out and move forward with a constant squeeze from both legs dropped to the back leg position. I will keep that squeeze (or increase the pressure) until he steps out or increases his forward movement. If I briefly kick and immediately release the squeeze he will believe I must have gotten the answer I was wanting. He figures whatever I wanted he must have given me the correct response. The brevity of many cues often works against the rider in clearly communicating what they want from their horse. The kick may work with some reactionary horses in getting a startled, forward movement, but it's purely coincidental.

By Anita J Howe

To truly communicate your wishes you need to keep squeezing until he moves off and then immediately release your squeeze when you get the desired forward movement. In this way your horse learns the squeeze in

Release is where the horse learns!

Release is by far the MOST important of the R's because it is the breakthrough moment when a horse finds the right answer and we get to tell him "YES! That's what I want!" release and reward his effort. Until we release our horse has no clear idea what we want of him. All of his responses are just guessing until we tell him "Yes" by releasing the cue. For this reason release is vital to training any horse.

Every rider should learn to perfect RELEASE if you wish to be a successful communicator with your horse. You should always try to *immediately give some kind of release* whenever you get a positive action from your horse and in this way strengthen his understanding of the correct and desired movement. I try to release and give a horse several seconds to absorb the fact that I released him and to enjoy his reward before beginning the sequence again for the next R of repetition.

Caution must be exercised not to inadvertently give release by mistake. Remember whatever your horse does just before you release him is what he will believe you want; that is what he will have learned is his correct. So if you inadvertently release your cue incorrectly it is very easy to teach a horse the wrong thing. I frequently see people honestly teaching their horses to misbehave by not being careful about when they release quite unintentionally. One of the most common things unintentionally taught behaviors is when a horse tosses his head, unhappy with either the bit or the hands on the reins. The rider ignores the head tossing until the horse gets even more strenuous with his objection, finally even lifting up off his front hooves

the back position means move forward or go faster forward. You can then apply this same squeeze or pressure in a forward position to move backward, and suddenly you're having a dialogue with your horse.

in a small rearing action. Boy that gets the attention of the rider and as the horse rears up the rider freaks out and releases the reins to grab the horn for stability. *This rider just taught his horse to rear up.* Yep, every time rider takes a hold on the reins this horse is going to remember the last time he got release when he reared, so he'll eventually go there again, and the more often he is successful in gaining his release he will go there faster and faster. Now this horse is labeled a problem or even dangerous horse because he's learned to always try this response when he's uncomfortable in his mouth.

What the rider should have done is release one rein only and pull this horse's head around to their knee, keeping the head as low as he can reach and holding him until he calms and settles. Only when the horse calms and gets release can the rider progress to find out why their horse was tossing his head in the first place. Don't ignore an action such as head tossing, tail swishing or stomping. This horse is trying to communicate a serious discomfort. Even if an action on the reins is what caused inadvertent discomfort to the horse, he must have no doubt that rearing, kicking or bucking is NEVER tolerated without correction. If you have a rearing horse, first look for a mouth problem: too severe of a bit, too heavy on the reins with a rider's hands or even bad teeth may be likely culprits.

REPETITION: The fourth and final R is just what it says. Once you have established a successful cycle of training above, wait a few moments then repeat the entire sequence. Repetition is what cements the horse's response into his memory. Typically the first

70

few correct responses are tentative, but by the time you've repeated 8 or 10 more times the horse is getting it. Make sure you don't burn them out. I get a dozen good responses, then move on to something else and come back to it later for a couple of quick refresher cues. If he can remember it after moving to something else then coming back, you've got it!

Some cues are so important that we need to repeat every day until a horse's response becomes ingrained and automatic; a conditioned response. We need to breech the thinking moment and train him to give a particular response so automatically it is like Pavlov's dogs. The one rein stop is just such a cue, so please read the following section on this critical tool. Every horse we hope to ride on the trail should be trained to calm and slow with the one rein stop. No matter how excited, worried or frightened a horse becomes, we need him to be so conditioned to the one rein stop that he will react by coming down to calmness and into thinking mode simply by pulling his nose to our calf. The one rein stop is as close to an emergency break as you can have on any horse, and by the way, you don't have to have a curb bit to do it!

Chapter 7 – Bit Training

The greatest gift you can give your horse and yourself is to train him to softly follow the bit.

*B*it training is both an investment in, as well as a kindness to, your horse. Contrary to popular belief, the bit should never be considered a brake or a steering wheel. It is *A SUBTLE TOOL* to be used to direct, instruct, and at times to contain forward energy. It is your tool to communicate to your horse how you would like him to carry his head and sometimes to direct him in focusing his energy. No horse should ever leave the training arena until you have him *LISTENING AND RESPONSIVE TO LIGHT BIT COMMUNICATION*. I simply cannot stress this enough. A bit should never be used to create pain or discomfort, nor to consistently control a horse, but for communication and direction of how we wish the horse to carry the area of his body in front of his shoulders.

CONNECTION NOT CONTACT

I've actually been accused by a few dressage enthusiasts of *THROWING AWAY CONTACT WITH MY HORSE* when I reward by releasing bit pressure. I guess it all depends on your definition of contact. It is my belief that riding with contact should be **no constant direct pressure on the bit**. None. I hold the reins where I'm supporting only their weight just an inch or so away from making that direct taut contact with the bit. I do this by holding them between thumb and forefinger then using my lower three fingers to collect the reins for contact or release them for reward.

Rather than contact, I prefer to call this riding with connection through the bit and reins. If you have doubt that this is active communication with your horse, hold a bit in your hands in front of your body while someone stands behind you with the reins, then have them jiggle or flutter one rein with no actual taut contact on the bit and feel how much life you can easily sense without that actual hard contact. This is just with our hands. Then imagine how sensitive the horse is when he's carrying that steel bit with his delicate mouth.

With bit training you must always be conscious of the potential for easily sliding into abusive pressure. Bit work is a responsibility as well as a slippery slope. It doesn't take much to cross the line when we're working with hard steel on a soft mouth tissue. We should always encourage our horse to listen to the bit with lightness and he will do this better if he has learned to trust the comfort and lightness of your bit connection. Much like we listen closer when someone whispers, the horse will listen closer to our communications if we whisper with our hands. Conversely, just as we will tend to shut out someone who is yelling or argumentative, a horse will shut down and tune out a rider who is nagging, harsh and abusive with their bit connection. This is what occurs when horses get hard in their mouth. They are shutting us out as best they can and ignoring the pressure to the best of their ability. I sure cannot imagine preferring to ride a horse like this.

Another byproduct of riding with constant bit pressure is the bit/reins/hands may well become a crutch to your horse. Horses often

WHERE TO START

Do yourself a favor and begin the basics of bit training from the ground with the lateral gives in a side-pull or a rope halter. This foundation helps your horse understand the basic lesson that we wish him to move *with* pressure; giving him the opportunity to learn this important lesson in a gentler manner. My philosophy is that bit communication is always a case of *LESS IS BETTER* as long as the horse is responsive. But it takes practice and a certain amount of self discipline to ride while allowing the horse the freedom of his head >90% of the time. It also takes practice to learn to communicate subtly with lightness and release.

Note: during lessons and clinics I frequently instruct riders to whisper to their horses. *"Always start every cue with a whisper before even considering increasing your volume toward a shout for that is the only way to develop a light and responsive horse"*. I illustrate this by whispering to say "see how you listen harder when someone speaks softly?" The same thing happens with our horses. As we lighten with our legs and hands they start listening more carefully. If you never try to cue lighter your horse will always remain stiff, and sluggish in his responses. It is only through softer cues that he will learn to listen closer and respond lighter. This is

start leaning into that pressure and using it to balance themselves. When a horse balances on the bit, he relies on the pressure to carry his gait and his self carriage is compromised. If or when he stumbles or missteps he will have a more difficult time recovering his balance. His athleticism is compromised in this posture. Also they start believing that they can only gait when they are leaning on the bit. This belief takes your horse down a path where the more he leans into the bit the greater the tension, the more he goes dorsally dominant, pacier and stiffer throughout his topline.

never more true than with bit training. When wielding the reins attached to a steel bit in the mouth of your horse you NEVER want to shout, so patience and persistence becomes even more important.

Reining enthusiasts understand the philosophy of relying more on seat and legs while preserving the bit for more important and subtle cues. Gaited riders, on the other hand, are notorious for mistakenly thinking they must frame up the horse into a head-set (grimace). In my opinion headset should be considered a four letter word. Rather than frame up headset, I believe in asking for correct head carriage then *RELEASING* the horse into self carriage. Carriage is something to be asked for by the rider and offered by the horse. We want our gaited horses to be encouraged to freely nod their heads productively at the flatfoot walk, the running walk and the foxtrot. We want them to travel in balance and athleticism, with lightness on the fore. So why then would we want to bind up their head and inhibit these very actions by framing their headset?

Let me stress one important point here. When you apply force to *ANY PART* of a horse, the horse reacts with natural tension, bracing and resistance unless you train him to give. If there is one overriding theme to this book it is to train your horse to give to pressure, to follow the bit and move off the leg without resistance and with the confident reassurance that your cue will be released as soon as he does. This means investing your time in training your horse to the four R's of Request, Response, Release and Repetition… patiently teaching them to follow and give to whatever cue or pressure you apply.

So if your horse is totally ignoring your cue, don't get mad and don't up the ante through force. Learn to **be patient and persistent**; to be annoying rather than abusive. Be the fly that won't go away until he gives. Relax yourself and basically say to him *"I can do this all day long if that's what it takes…."* But always be ready to release him and reward him as soon as he *gets it*.

This does not mean that lighter is always better. While I generally would far prefer to see a rider being too light rather than too harsh with a bit, I have seen a few instances when a rider seems almost afraid to make connection, repetitively fluttering a bit that their horse is quite happily ignoring. This is the case of too light and too frequent cues producing more of a static noise rather than a confident, solid asking cue. Ideally we want a mild bit that the horse can learn to be comfortable carrying coupled with an easy tug and hold cue, releasing only upon getting the desired response from the horse (The 4 R's). If the horse ignores you, you will need *to increase the range motion while never yanking or jerking*. A controlled bend or tug, at first ignored, can be increased in motion without getting abusive where the motion is increased in a controlled manner. For instance, starting with a one-rein half-halt, when ignored can be deliberately increased into greater bend and eventually into a full turn for disengagement of the hind quarters when the horse fails to respond. When the horse learns to respond you can then get lighter and lighter with your asking cue and in this way he learns to listen and respond to those light asking cues.

Never let yourself be lured to going bigger with the bit if you cannot get the desired movement with less at first. It's quite common that when a horse just doesn't seem to **get it** that someone will come along to tell you to get a more serious bit. Some professional trainers and a even few clinicians may advocate this notion. But I will only recommend moving to a curb bit when your horse is light and responsive in a snaffle and even then NEVER using curb bit with shanks longer than 6 inches. If your horse gets stiff or resistant, you need to go back to the snaffle to re-train and soften him, not the other way around. Much like spurs, you should earn the right to use more severe bitting only as your horse has graduated in his responsiveness. It never fails that when I suggest you don't need longer shanks, someone will chime in to say *"any bit can be abusive in the wrong hands"* and they are technically correct. My response to that is "what does a 10 inch shank give you that you cannot achieve with a 5 inch shank or even a snaffle for that matter?" I will never advocate going to a more severe bit when you are unsuccessful with a milder one. Instead *you* need to get better with less. It's possible that you are progressing faster than your horse is ready to, and you may need back up and refresh the basic maneuvers, get lighter and lighter at those movements and only then progress into more complex challenges. Sometimes this simply means slowing down or taking a few moments to refreshing some cues at a stop. Sometimes you may need to break down the desired movement into smaller baby steps that are more manageable and more easily understood. A more severe bit will invariably cause your horse to lose his lightness and become more stiff in his movement even if you do manage to get the short term goal accomplished.

In the following sections you will find instruction on what I consider six essential movements of the head and neck to be asked for by you and given or offered by your horse. All of these should be trained initially at a standstill, and then re-taught at the walk. Some will also come become very useful for modifying gait. If you can accomplish a light and willing responsiveness from your horse with these movements you should never need to resort to a harsher bit to control your horse. If ever the horse later does become stiff and resistant, you simply go back to the drawing board and refresh. I advocate starting every ride by running through this series of bit exercises or movements before you ever ask your horse to walk out. Much like a runner will stretch before he takes off, you should offer your horse the opportunity of a refresher before you start out on your rides.

THE SIX MOVEMENTS

In order to have a great working partnership and make the most of this important tool of changing how the horse carries his head and neck, we must be able to ask and the horse give us **SIX BASIC MOVEMENTS** and postures with his head. I will list them here in progression that I recommend you use to train them.

TOOLS: I highly recommend that you consider using a snaffle bit (direct action) to simplify this training process. The snaffle will give your horse a much better opportunity to be successful. If you're not comfortable working with a snaffle, you might try starting with it in a very enclosed area such as the round pen. I've even had green horses that I've used a large foaling stall to start their bit training. However if you truly do not want to climb onto your horse without the action of a curb, please be mindful that when you use a curb you must be lighter than ever with your cues and must be more patience in allowing him time to figure out the movements you are wanting.

I also recommend using a sport or roping rein or even an English rein if you have it. This single rein gives YOU less to worry about; allows you to focus more on your horse and less on keeping split reins together and sliding evenly. I personally prefer a 10 foot sport rein. The traditional roper reins are only 7 ½ to 8 feet long and for larger horses you will find that length somewhat limiting as he drops his head low. The normal 11 to 12 feet of the mecate reins are really a little excessive and the excess becomes somewhat cumbersome to deal with. Nine to ten feet is almost the perfect length for most average size horses. I also like the softer braided cotton or marine rope reins for repetitive sliding through your hands without chafing.

It is **IMPORTANT** that you begin training these movements while *at a standstill*. It becomes an entirely different movement once the horse's feet are moving forward. Find a place where your horse is comfortable, and he is willing to stand calmly. When his feet are not moving he listens better. Being stopped isolates your cues to just his head, allowing you to keep your legs and seat in a neutral, released posture and thereby reducing the potential for confusion. Once he understands a cue and becomes consistent with his correct response, you can begin to walk him slowly forward and re-teach that cue at the walk, later at gait and later still at the canter. Establish a consistent response at the stop and slow walk before progressing faster.

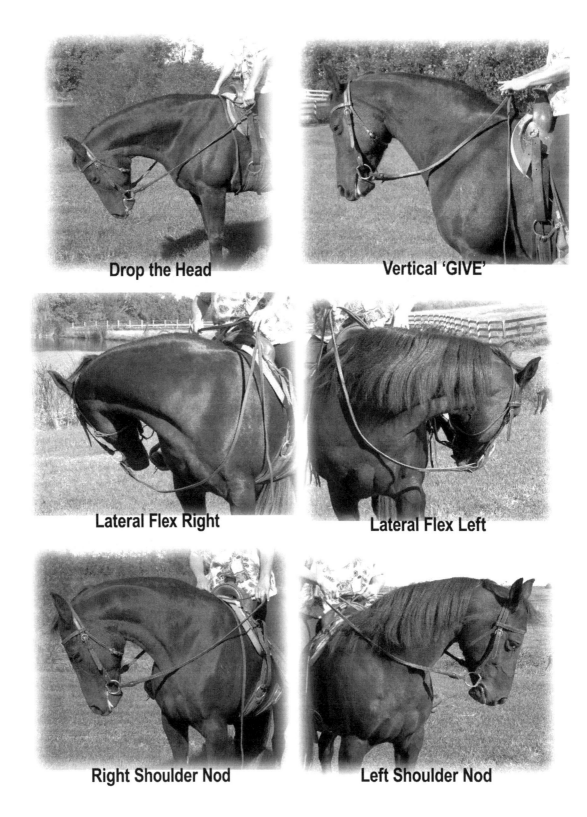

Figure 7.1 Papa's Graceful Spirit

LATERAL FLEX (RIGHT AND LEFT)

This basic bit movement is popular with just about every natural horseman out there. Apply light pressure on one rein, pulling it toward your knee or thigh while always making certain the opposite rein totally released with slack. Hold and pause while waiting for the horse's response. Remember ***know what you want before you begin.*** The desired response should be a slight give by your horse in the direction of the rein pressure creating slack in that pulling rein. Be extra careful to keep your legs off the horse's sides. It is important that you do not unintentionally give him mixed signals. If using a single roper or sport rein use the opposite hand to hold it in a centered position or at the buckle. If you're using split reins hold both reins at a slack with that off hand while pulling with your active hand. This positioning of hands and rein will allow you to release the cue pressure **the instant** you feel your horse give toward your leg, while maintaining hold of the reins with the off hand. This is a practiced move that Clinton Anderson is very good at demonstrating in his training videos. It is important to maintain a balanced and independent seat so that if the horse circles (and most do at first) you are ready for it and do not change the cue in response to his shift in position.

Apply steady rein pressure lightly and consistently while holding until you see his effort to give, then the *QUICKER YOU CAN RELEASE* all pressure (and I do mean totally release and drop the rein from that hand) the quicker the horse can begin to understand that he gave you the right answer. He needs to make the mental connection between his give to your release. The first couple of times most horses will begin to get a glimmer or beginning to understand. After 5 or 6 positive responses and releases the light bulb is beginning to glow. After a dozen the horse has realized it's a game that he can play and most do so quite willingly. Both

directions must be established, and I advise alternating sides at *IRREGULAR* repetitions to avoid the horse trying to anticipate rather than truly listening to what you are asking.

RESISTANCE: If your horse shows a stiffness to one side or other (and most of them do at first) you must work the bend on that side a little more regularly until he becomes equally soft and flexible side-to-side. It is important to remember that if a horse is bending and giving correctly you should see a nice *ARCHING CURVE* to his neck as he bends. If he's stiff he may resist the give completely at first then when he does bend you may notice most of the actual bend happening at the base of his neck and at his poll, while the rest of his neck appears pretty straight. You may also notice his nose will tend to push out and his poll will try to elevate. This is a resistant posture that indicates he's stiff and needs to learn to give *BY BRINGING HIS CHIN IN TOWARD YOUR LEG, AND LOWER BOTH HIS POLL AND HIS ENTIRE NECKLINE.* His chin should remain at or around the level of the point of his shoulder and come toward your foot. If it is higher he is probably showing some resistance because he's not as supple as he needs to be. The bend exercise IS the cure for this stiffness, you just need to be aware of his potential stiffness and ask for this bend slowly but persistently while keeping your active rein hand down near your calf. Lead his nose down where you need it to be. As the horse gives the offside muscles are the ones that must stretch and release in his neck, so any side that shows resistance is evidence of tight, unconditioned muscles on the opposite side of his neck. Working the lateral give slowly but persistently should help your horse soften and loosen his neck as well as learning to follow your bit pressure.

This right and left lateral give to-the-leg represents the first two bit movements to train. After working both sides of this exercise move on to something else for a little while then come back to the bit training. Give a refresher

Drop-the-head

This movement is a wonderful tool that allows you to communicate at what level you wish your horse to carry his head and neck, as well as to encourage him to stretch out his topline between vigorous collected movements and exercises. I always release my horses into a long and low stretch as reward and to encourage calm down. I have taught many, many horses to drop the head from a variety of different cues. The cue I chose for a particular horse will sometimes depend on the riding style of the owner, or sometimes because a horse simply responds to one cue better than the other. My initial and preferred cue is a two handed stretch-into-the-bit cue.

Again this works best with English or roper reins where you can place both hands on the rein, sliding them apart and down until your forearms are resting on or near your thighs. You should be applying a *LIGHT BUT CONSTANT* downward tug on the bit. It is important to understand that we need only about 2- 4 ounces of pressure with a mild snaffle. Anything greater may cause the horse to brace and push back or to lean on the bit with resistance. Our goal is to not to cause discomfort, just to be annoying so the horse does not ignore us. I apply this pressure, remaining relaxed while *CAREFULLY WATCHING THE POLL BY FOCUSING MY EYES* between the ears (any place high on the head will do, this is just where I focus). At first it is quite typical for horses to ignore the pressure. Once the horse

few lateral gives to each side and do so again at the beginning of each daily ride.

starts moving his head it's almost as if he's saying "what do you want?" When it does not go away or lessen, they will begin moving their head around to test that pressure. They may push against it, try going side to side, and/or lifting. All of which you will ignore as you patiently wait for his correct response which is any downward movement. Remember you don't want to release to his wrong answer so be patient. As soon as he makes *ANY* downward motion IMMEDIATELY drop the reins loose. Pause for a moment to let him think about what just happened and repeat.

As your horse advances in his practice of this movement you can use it to go lower and lower. I feel a horse finally **gets it** when he's willing to stretch all the way to the ground, and sometimes even reward him by dropping a treat on the ground for him to reach for so that it becomes more of a game. As I instruct in the FOUR R'S OF TRAINING, from here you need to repeat until you can get a consistently correct response. I would further advise that when you are getting a repeatable response, you give the horse a break to avoid him become sour about any lesson. Come back a short while later and do a few more drop-the-head movements just to make certain he remembers then put it away for the day. At this point it should become part of your daily warm up routine along with other yielding and bending cues. This becomes your third movement of bit training.

Vertical Give

Where the drop-the-head cue is working to get the entire head and neck column to lower allowing the nose to reach toward the ground, the vertical give is a similar but essentially different movement. Most of the

flexion of the drop-the-head occurs at the base of the neck. The vertical give focuses much more on the poll. We do not necessarily want the horse to lower his head so much, but we'll not penalize that movement either. We want a poll flexion along with a rounding of the neck while bringing the chin toward his chest.

I recommend using what I term a bit flutter to cue and ask for the vertical give. **PLEASE do not saw at the horse's mouth.** This should be a light and subtle, alternating *fingertip flutter or waggle* that is not uncomfortable, just a little annoying for the horse. It is a light action using only your fingertips, never your wrists, and certainly never moving your elbows. You may even allow drape and looseness to remain in the reins once you start getting a repeatable response from your horse because by then he knows what you're wanting and he's listening for it.

Again, as with the drop the head, you lightly continue the cue while watching closely and patiently for the horse's correct response, and as soon as you see or feel even a slight give at the poll, you immediately drop the reins loose, quit the cue for several moments as a reward and release for the horse. Because the horse's nose is usually straight in front of his neckline it may be more difficult to see the desired response when it happens. So you need to look for two things: the reins to go slack as he moves his nose toward his chest if you have your hands stable and your arms anchored his correct movement will create slack in the reins. Another thing to watch for is the muscles just below the poll on each side of his neck. These will widen or bulge as he flexes his poll.

Be happy at first with a slight give and looseness in the rein, but continue to work the movement until you can flutter his chin very close to his chest. This is NOT a continuously braced position to be held in like the Rollkur, but an ask-and-release movement and exercise that pays tremendous dividends as a tool for gait alteration.

This becomes the fourth movement of bit training and like all the rest should be added to your daily start up stretching routine.

THE SHOULDER NOD

Here we want a movement that has characteristics of both the lateral bend and the vertical give. Our goal is for the horse to 'nod' his chin toward the point of his shoulder with a single light pull on one rein, though we may have to utilize both reins in a supporting manner to help him find this movement initially. It becomes a very important tool as we progress in training for leg yields. You're looking for a lighter lateral bend through the neck coupled with a give at the poll that rounds his neckline forward. *IT WILL APPEAR THAT THE HORSE IS ALMOST TOUCHING HIS CHIN TO HIS SHOULDER*, his poll toward 1 o'clock on the right or 11 o'clock on the left.

While I do not work this movement as much at a standstill it is invaluable as a starting point for the above mentioned walking movements. It also significantly promotes softness to the neckline that will aid the lift of the lower neck that is so important in front-to-back balance.

People watching me train will note that I frequently use this tool to aid in rebalancing and bringing a horse back into softness at a walking speed. As with all the bit cues I teach and use, it is always to be asked for, NEVER forced. As soon as a horse gives it *WE SHOULD ALWAYS RELEASE AND REPEAT UNTIL HE LEARNS TO CARRY IT OR HOLD IT.* As he progresses with his training, often a quick tug on one rein is all you'll need for him to immediately soften and drop his backend down into engagement in a rebalancing motion as he gives this movement and lifts his lower neck.

I begin training this very simply, but with great patience. A light pull on one rein to bring the head to the one o'clock position on the right or the eleven o'clock position on the left. You pull the rein to this point, anchor your forearm against your thigh, then wait and watch closely. This is your eventual finished cue and all you will need once the horse has learned, so we want to always begin with this action. If you have followed my example of cues for both lower-the-head and the vertical give so far then you'll note that this cue, like the movement itself, is a combination of both. After a short moment of holding the above light lateral flexion ask you should pick up the outside rein and give light flutter (stress the word *light*) while reaching that hand down in a much lower position that will encourage the horse's chin to drop and his neck to round as it does in the vertical give. This takes a little practice on your part and, again, you should train it while stopped because reaching this low may compromise your balance in the saddle initially if you're not used to it. Be ready again for your horse to begin circling in his search to understand what you're asking. Eventually you'll not need this supporting rein as your horse becomes more polished at this movement. It is important that you have the vertical give very well established before you

begin training this shoulder nod.

You want to see the horse bring his chin toward his shoulder while flexing at the poll and rounding his entire neckline. The right and left shoulder nods represent the final two of our six bit training movements.

These six bit movements give you the dialogue with your horse to ask him to carry his head in just about any position you need or feel will help him at any moment or gait. As such they are, in my opinion, just as essential as the reins and bit to training the naturally gaited horse. Always remember that you want to ask your horse for head and neck positioning and never brace or hold in. It is so imperative that your horse understand that when and if you take hold of the bit you want him to change something. You should never just hold on to keep him somewhere. That erroneous thinking is why we end up with stiff, locked and unbalanced gaited horses. Ask, give and release are all terms of a willing partnership.

ONE REIN STOP

The one rein stop is an essential training tool that I feel every horse needs in his repertoire. It is as close to a brake as can be established with any horse. In my opinion the one rein stop (ORS) is a *MUST* for any horse before he leaves the training arena. It should be established so completely and thoroughly that no matter what spooks him on the trail, whether it's a bicycle, a deer or a mountain lion, you need to have the tool to bring him mentally back to you, and the ORS is just such a tool.

Choose an open area where your horse can easily circle on groomed level ground. Begin training the ORS at a *SLOW WALKING SPEED*, sliding one hand down arm's length on the rein and pulling that rein to your knee. It is important to keep the drawing motion low toward your knee, because a higher head angle on the horse's bend will jam his neck and create discomfort that could actually

make him more afraid and spooky. If you have properly trained the lateral gives, your horse should be acceptable to this movement.

You hold this rein to your knee while your horse usually begins circling at first. Be prepared for this circle by moving your opposite stirrup slightly away from the horse to brace your weight shift in that direction. Relax and be patient, making certain to keep your legs off his sides while you watch for him to do two things: stop moving his feet and give to the bit with a light nod in the direction of your knee creating a moment of looseness in the rein. Train this cue in an enclosed arena and practice first at a slow walking speed, then at the flatfoot walk, then intermediate gaiting speed.

The ORS is **NOT** to be used when a horse is moving at full gallop speed in a bolting action. In those situations you need to learn to slow him by circling large. As he begins to slow down continue to spiral him into smaller and smaller circles and eventually into a one rein stop. If you tried to execute a one rein stop with a horse at a full bolt or gallop, the bending to your knee would likely cause him to unbalance and both of you go rolling at high speed. Very ugly, risky and unnecessary. Bend him into a large circle – don't panic – tighten the circle as he slows so he can maintain his balance – don't panic - then go into a full ORS from this slower speed. Above all Don't

Panic! You must be thinking and not reacting, just as we want your horse to start thinking and not reacting.

Don't wait to try this for the first time during a moment of emergency. Practice this maneuver first in the round pen, then in the arena and finally in an open field. The ORS is your safety, your panic switch, your emergency break. At least as much as ANY horse can have an emergency break.

UNDERSTANDING THE HALF-HALT

I believe the half-halt evolved from a need to release a horse into *CORRECT* movement, even though this may not be the classical explanation taught. Releasing into action is particularly appropriate when the desired movement is one of fluid balance and impulsion, which most athletic maneuvers should be. The process of releasing the horse encourages him, but in order to release we first must apply brief pressure or resistance to his current movement. Riders have found that a short capture of the horse's energy through the bit connection and supported with the seat encourages him to hesitate just long enough to gather himself. When that capture is then immediately released and followed with a light-to-moderate driving aid to ask for impulsion we find the horse can apply this gathered energy with more precision and balance. So you see half-halts regularly used to ask the horse both to rebalance and to prepare for balanced action.

You most likely will not be able to get a green or untrained horse to pay attention to the subtle cue that a true half-halt should be. So don't be disappointed if you try it on your horse and he totally ignores you at first. You have to train the horse to get lighter and listen closer to rein and seat cues to get full benefit from the half-halt or the one-rein half-halt. This means being patient and persistent in

training your horse to understand what you're wanting.

I think what I want to stress here is that a half-halt is a method of communication that should always be light and subtle. I believe our goal should always be to keep the vast majority of rein communication, including the half-halt, as a light communication from our fingertips *KEEPING OUR ELBOWS AND WRISTS QUIET*. When I need to signal the horse to gather, to rebalance or to alter his falling out of balance, I give a quick fingertip tug more to resist his incorrect motion than to completely interrupt his flow. Sometimes during the training process you may even see a half-halt used to warn the horse that he needs to gather himself better or a correction will soon follow. As the horse progresses the half-halts can become lighter and more of a quiet cue to rebalance and less as a warning. The half-halt is an invaluable tool for all these uses.

Lightness becomes even more important when we desire very forward movement that we do not wish to interrupt. For instance when I wish to keep a horse moving forward and not discourage his reach or stride I have found a **ONE REIN HALF-HALT** is often even more effective than the more traditional two-handed half-halt. My experience is that when you grab both reins even for a very brief moment, it creates the proverbial wall in the horse's mouth. This wall will invariably cause the horse to shorten his forward reach and is particularly troublesome when working with walking horses that I wish to encourage their reach to maximize their stride. That wall becomes counterproductive to my goals and desires for this horse. How then can I signal him to gather or rebalance himself without creating this wall of resistance? Rather than grabbing with both hands, I've learned to tug and release with one rein only, usually supported by a quick hug of my calf on that same side so that it almost becomes a very light (or really just the threat of) a leg yield or bend. This supporting calf pressure also encourages him to continue traveling straight rather than follow any bend of his nose. It is, in fact, a half-halt with a driving aid. I train the horse first that if he chooses to ignore this brief signal, I will continue this movement into a full bend. This quick one-rein tug then evolves into both a request for him to rebalance and a warning not to ignore my request or he will end up in a complete bending circle. I found that the one rein half-halt was even lighter and quicker cue than the two handed half-halt that is traditionally taught. The one rein cue can be very slow and deliberate, taking a full (one-thousand-one)second for resist-and-release or a very brief flutter depending on how closely the horse is listening to me and at what stage his training is at.

Some will argue that by using only one hand I am unbalancing the horse or causing him NOT to travel with straightness. This is not the case if you have taught your horse to travel straight by following your LEGS and to understand that the reins are not to redirect him but to instruct how he should carry his head and neck only. If he has successfully learned this the supporting pressure of my calf on the same side keeps the horse traveling straight and true. I would also argue that the inherent stiffness found in many of the gaited breeds benefits from the added bend and suppleness which traveling through the shoulder or through the bend can add. The horse naturally wants to travel straight and I will reward and encourage that straightness as long as it is correct straightness.

All of the bit training we discuss above can and should evolve into subtle cues that become lighter and lighter as your horse progresses in his training allowing you get lighter and lighter in the way you ask. A horse should graduate to less interruption as he improves and soon all you need is a light reminder action when he begins to lose balance or fall into an undesired gait. These are the mechanics of the half-halt and however you desire to implement it you should always try to do so with lightness and subtlety.

RIDING BACK TO FRONT

Gait doesn't *HAPPEN* in the head any more than it *HAPPENS* in the feet. People often get so preoccupied with the headnodding movement for the walking gaits and the foxtrot they start believing that if they can just get the head motion the gait will be correct or better.

It is critical to understand that head and neck motion (or lack thereof) is *AN EXPRESSION* of what the body is doing. *IT IS A PRODUCT OF GAIT, AND NOT THE SOURCE OF GAIT.* The misconception that "if I can just get the headnod I'll have a horse walking (or foxtrotting)" is what leads people to try to force a particular movement through the bit with their hands. I've even heard some claim they time up a horse through his mouth referring to the isochronal timing of his legs. You frequently see people bumping, pumping and tweaking on those reins being very rude to their horse and thinking it's all about what they're doing with their hands, and they couldn't be more wrong. I see this a great deal with folks who have been training their gaited horses for years, so this tells me how prevalent this misconception is within both the walking horse and the foxtrot world. There is some limited success to it, but you are far too often sabotaging your horse's balance by trying to force a motion from the head backward. Not to mention how uncomfortable he must be with a rider being so rude to his mouth.

It is of interest that one of the arguments brought forth during the FEI discussion regarding the use of Rollkur in competition states

1 - A system of riding that works from hindquarters --->> toward the bridle is logically and biomechanically sound.

2 - A system of riding that works from forequarters toward the hindquarters <u>contradicts the structures of the horse.</u>

In summation: get the gait and the headnod will follow - kind of an "if you build it he will come" situation. When a horse gives you the head position you ask for, you must release his mouth so he can carry that gait. True brilliance with correct head usage comes from the confident freedom of his head and being allowed to express all the energy and action coming from both the driving backend

and the reaching, rolling shoulder. Misapplied rein contact will inhibit this natural brilliance and more often degrade the gait rather than help it. So reward your horse with the freedom to give you the gait you're looking for and stay out of his mouth as much as possible.

Likewise dressage instructors who have no experience with gaited horses may try to instruct you on how to maintain contact with your horse while riding, and that advice may very well be more detrimental to your riding partnership than beneficial. This is why I strongly advocate **connection rather than contact**. You need to learn to release your horse into gait by using a half-halt and release. This rewards your horse for correct carriage and significantly reduces the risk of mistakenly introducing tension into the equation by framing the bit with constant contact. It further makes this correct carriage more comfortable for your horse which also encourages him to want to be there. If you never fully release the bit your horse feels there is no reward for him in learning correct self carriage because you have taken away his incentive.

Chapter 8 —Power Steering for Your Horse

I illustrated earlier that to truly create a partnership with your horse you should develop a method of communicating with him. Every one of the celebrity trainers actively working the expos and the TV programming has a method they have perfected and are teaching to others. You will naturally observe similarities in their methods, but differences as well. In this chapter I discuss my method of riding and communicating with gaited horses to work to improve their balance, softness and impulsion in those key areas that will make them a better riding horse and enable us to help them alter, improve and condition their gaits naturally.

To preserve the respect and trust of your horse you need to ride using less hands by using more seat and legs. Understanding that the bit is not there to stop the horse, nor really even to steer the horse, but only to help him understand how we want him to carry everything in front of his legs is essential. From there his trust is preserved by teaching release, release, release of the bit and hands. Let your

horse carry himself in balanced self carriage without you trying to hold him, pull him in or frame him into gait. One of my favorite sayings is that *without self carriage your horse cannot have self balance, and without correct self balance HIS ATHLETICISM will be compromised.* So let's let him balance himself and learn to self carry to maintain his athleticism by trying to never unnecessarily pull on his head.

The point to all of all this is to encourage you to always be aware of contact with your horse. If you constantly have to steady your balance using your hands you are continually being rude to his mouth and inhibiting your horse's balance. Give him the respect of releasing his head and mouth until you have reason not to. In this manner your horse begins to understand that when you do make contact you are asking for him to change and he will listen and pay closer attention to that contact. Further your goal should be to always try to direct the movement of his feet first with your own legs and seat.

RIDING POSITION

To have confidence in riding with less hand contact, you need to not only have better balance in your seat but learn better ways to communicate direction and speed to your horse without the reins. A deeper, steadier seat with calmer, less dramatic hand

movements both helps you stay balanced and be more precise in your communications with your horse. Utilizing the three leg positions can give you exactly that kind of language for communicating everything you wish your horse to do from his shoulders back.

Your balance is the foundation of learning to ride with less rein contact. I encourage people to ride with deep stirrups to improve their balance as well as to better communicate with their legs. If you can reach under and below the horse's midpoint on his sides (a real advantage for long legged riders) you can apply a lifting calf pressure low on his ribs. This is a huge tool in helping him understand when we wish him to lift his shoulders and lower neck. If you can use your calf muscles to hug and lift near the girth he will soon start to understand you wish him to lighten in this area. Every horse is different but you might be surprised at how quickly your horse picks up on this. Another tremendous benefit to riding with deeper stirrups is *the lower you position your legs and arms the lower your center of gravity becomes.* The lower your center of balance, the more secure and solid you will be in the saddle. Those riders who sit perched upon their horse with their arms raised even with or higher than their elbows are way more top heavy and are less secure in their balance. Riding with deep stirrups while keeping your hands and arms low against your sides aids in placing your center of balance nearer and deeper into the saddle. *This significantly steadies you in the event of a side jump or startle.* Also learning to grip the saddle from knee to knee will add steadiness as well as support, while providing you the option of circling your heels in and hugging the horse to reinforce your balance. Your stirrups should be adjusted no higher than ankle length when you hang your legs straight down. This stirrup length gives you just enough support to balance and lift yourself out of the saddle for brief moments if needed while encouraging a deep leg posture.

Besides an overall balanced seat you need the ability to use your seat and legs with strength and coordination. I will admit this takes some practice and you'll certainly build those glutes in learning to ride more with strong legs. But aside from buns of steel you'll

also learn to communicate with your horse in a way that allows him to stay confident while trusting that you're serious about holding up your side of the contract.

I am not a fan of the chair seat positioning that is advocated by some gaited clinicians and the saddleseat equitation as a whole. Nor does the hypothesis that 'if we ride bareback with our legs forward it must be best' hold water for me. When riding bareback you completely forfeit the use of the stirrups for balancing, which takes away any triangulation of your balance, and naturally you move your knees forward to compensate for this lack. I do ride bareback with my legs more forward for that very reason, but when I have stirrups, I drop my heels back into equitation position because that is the most balanced and versatile position from which to both ride and cue the horse. Far too many people using a chair seat posture will tend to lean back placing greater weight on the back of the saddle (which we discussed is not beneficial for your horse's carriage or gait) and often offset this backward lean by hanging on the reins to balance themselves through the horse's mouth. This is VERY rude to your horse and a complete rejection of your responsibility to the partnership. The three leg positions below will be much easier and fluid if you lower your heels back under your seat cheeks. This placement helps tilt your pelvis forward to keep you centered, and makes dropping into the back leg position much easier.

- The forward position is near the girth line (even occasionally in front when trying to exaggerate and help the horse understand).
- The center position is directly beneath your seat, in equitation positioning with heels aligned below your shoulders.
- The back position is reaching BEHIND your seat, a little closer to his flank area.

The one consistent theme is to teach your

horse *TO MOVE AWAY FROM PRESSURE*. This should be established from the ground first with hand pressure making the transition to leg pressure in the saddle a natural evolution.

One leg applying pressure in forward position tells the horse to move his forelegs laterally in the opposite direction. Right leg pressure in forward position tells the horse to move his front legs laterally to the left. Your left leg in forward position means to step to the right. Your right leg in back position means to move his hindquarters to the left, and vice versa. Once you have the front and the back responding to single leg pressure you can begin training to pressure in the center position, which eventually will evolve to move

both front and back or to side pass.

Both legs in forward position with hugging pressure tells a horse to stop, slow forward movement or backup. Both legs applying light pressure in back position mean to increase forward speed or to walk out from a stop.

Using these basic pressure cues you can train your horse to move his legs in any direction. But probably your biggest challenge will be to remember and learn to ride this way. Practice supporting all bending, turning and movement of any kind with legs cues. You need to pay attention and learn, but once you begin to consistently use your legs, you can work the corners and train your horse to understand and respond lighter and lighter.

SEAT

This is a great moment to briefly explain about what I call your riding seat. I define your seat in three different modes: driving, passive and resisting. In learning to ride with more seat and less hands you need to communicate to your horse more actively than many of you are probably accustomed to.

The driving seat is an active movement that your horse can tell is asking for more. It is pushing, releasing, rolling of the hips and pelvis and overall a driving aid to encourage a greater energy output from him.

The passive seat is relaxed but moving with your horse's natural motions. The passive

seat isn't encouraging nor asking for more. The passive seat is not resisting or indicating a correction. You are telling your horse, through your seat that you like what he is doing and are happy for just this moment being a passenger. No pressure is being applied but you are happy to move WITH your horse's correct gait.

The resistant seat signals you do not like where he is at or where he is going with his movement. You wish to interrupt, to slow or to completely stop and you demonstrate this to your horse by tightening your thighs, bracing your lower back and resisting the natural movement of his gait.

WORKING THE CORNERS

Working the corners is an elementary schooling exercise that I start teaching my horses when first under saddle and still in the round pen. Until you have them responding to your legs, I do not advise you to leave the arena, let alone hit the open trails. Training the horse to your leg is a vital part of *putting the power steering on your horse* and should be part of foundation training for *any* horse.

Always work the corners from a stop.

Pick a leg: front or back on either side. Apply the opposite side pressure in the appropriate position, *HOLD AND WAIT FOR CORRECT MOVEMENT.* If there is no response at first slowly increase your leg pressure and use reins only to block forward walk-off movement or as added support. You're not trying to lead your horse in a circle, but get him to step to the side laterally with the desired leg. It is not unusual for a horse to try to walk off at the first application of even one leg pressure, and you'll need to use the reins to quickly and lightly block these attempts while giving light side directional support that is coordinated with your leg pressure. By directional support I mean the supporting rein should be against his neck while you ***open the door*** with the leading rein. Even if he shows no inclination to step away remember to keep the rein contact light since the entire purpose is to get him to respond to the leg cue first and foremost. Consequently always make certain to begin with the leg pressure first and use the rein only as needed if or when you get no response to the leg only. You apply the pressure, hold, wait and watch for the chosen leg to step laterally. Watch vigilantly and AS SOON AS YOU SEE THE DESIRED DIRECTION (EVEN A MINOR ATTEMPT) RELEASE ALL PRESSURE OF YOUR HAND AND LEG. Pause for reward. Repeat this same cue and direction until you are getting a repeatable response from the horse. Then move on to the next leg and repeat the process with each

leg of the horse. In this method you should be able to train your horse to move any of his legs laterally by how and where you apply pressure.

Eventually you'll be able to get a full 360 degree turn around all four corners of the horse built from this step-at-a-time progression. The back feet circle around the fore and the fore legs will create a haunch turn. This can be built into precise haunch and fore turns as you string together these steps for multiples and eventually to 180 and 360 degree turns. I make this a daily part of my training with novice horses right along with the bit training, since it is a vital part of keeping a horse between your legs and moving straight. The lateral movement off your leg is also the start of leg yields, diagonals and shoulders-in. Once you have reliably responsive movement for all four corners you can also begin working center position pressure with one leg for the side pass.

LESS HANDS MEANS BETTER BALANCE

Riding with less bit contact indicates commitment on the part of the rider and a sincere desire to establish a compatible partnership with the horse. It also demonstrates a desire to improve your riding ability and balance. Riding with less rein contact requires a more independent. As you learn to use the three leg positions and work the corners, your legs will get stronger and your balance will improve.

Many years ago a good friend and mentor,

Bruce Almeida, told me to ride a horse as though a wizard was going to "*wave a magic wand and make the horse disappear from beneath you at any moment. Balance when riding so that you will land and stand on your feet when the horse disappears."* This awareness immediately altered the way I was sitting in the saddle. It helped me balance over my heels and remain more centered as I rode. I pass this advice on with full confidence it can help anyone learn to have a more independent seat.

PATIENCE AND PERSISTENCE

If there is one most important thought that is worth restating about natural horsemanship it's that ***Horse training is 100% patience plus 100% persistence***. Remember that you're dealing with a creature who communicates non-verbally through body language, and you

need to learn to speak his language. To cross this language barrier takes a calm acceptance that it will not happen overnight, and while it's natural to feel frustration at times, if you ever get so tense that you cannot relax your face and whistle, it's time for a break. Look for the positives in every workout. Appreciate that these animals have both good and bad days just as we do, but as long as you feel they are willing and trying to play your game you should be happy. Find satisfaction in a journey that is both a challenge and a reward. Anything worth having is worth working for.

FIRST AND ALWAYS A HORSE

The idea that a gaited horse needs to be treated, ridden, tacked and cared for any differently than any other horse is plain silly. You should understand that a gaited horse is still a horse first, and should not treat him any differently than any other pleasure horse until you reach the point of polishing his gait. For the first six months under saddle I advise people to train them and start them just as they would any other horse breed. My only additional recommendation is to keep them to a walk for better muscle memory development.

Learning to ride a gaited horse is a lot like getting on a 21 speed mountain bike for the first time. Without some basic instruction most of us would probably fumble around until we find a gear or two that works OK, and settle for going about in those couple of speeds. But with a little information suddenly you find that you have all these gears (gaits) now available to you. Most gaited horses have multiple gaits available. They were bred for it.

I know there are folks within the gaited horse world who would have you believe that each breed should default into one set of bred-in gaits, find and use those gaits automatically without any specific knowledge or effort on the part of the rider. I am not in that camp. I just cannot believe that the founding breeders of these horses crossed hearty trotting breeds with fast and forward pacers with the intention of producing horses that would neither pace nor trot. I believe their intention was to produce horses that would find a multitude of gaits that could be utilized in a variety of situations. They wanted to produce a versatile horse more in line with the SUV's of the horse world. Horses that are able to cruise along with the Cadillac of rides on the groomed trail, road or across acres of plantation; go into 4 WD through the rugged hills, then pull the plows, pen the cows or draw the buggy as needed. It is my opinion that trying to insist these horses should be push button default one-gear gaiters requireing no particular skill or effort to ride does a disservice to these breeds and makes a one-sided glossy surface out of a diamond that should have multiple facets for real sparkle.

Those who would believe that the horses should be bred to default into one fixed gait find it all too easy to abandon any off-gaited horses as poorly bred and give up on them. I believe every one of these horses can learn to find an easy gait within their own conformational abilities, and to carry that smooth gait effortlessly within their own posture, balance and conditioning. I never want to give up on any horse.

Chapter 9 – Dressage for the Gaited Horse

A commonly accepted definition for dressage is *"the art of training a horse to be obedient and responsive to the rider"* and that certainly seems to encompass what most of us try to do though I would not consider myself a dressage trainer. The term dressage is normally used in referring to the English equestrian competition. I love to play with my horses and challenge them through dressage-type exercises because I believe it helps them learn to listen and helps me focus on what I'm asking them to do and how I go about it.

While I have taken dressage tests I do not define myself or my goals for my horses by those tests, unlike some. However, the longer I train horses the more I find myself utilizing these exercises for their specific benefit for a given horse. Some may say this is simply semantics, but though each exercise has a goal of striving for perfection, beyond those goals I've found benefits to the horses I'm working with. It is those benefits that have become my purpose behind the exercise, not the goal of perfection.

It is very important to note that some practices commonly accepted as part of this discipline are more difficult for gaited horses and you should be aware and consider these before attempting to ask your horse to engage himself this way. Many of the basic dressage exercises involve diagonal movements at a trot. While most gaited horses can be taught to find their trot, most gaited riders are hesitant to do so, and I can certain understand that. If you ask your horse to move in a diagonal direction while in gait he may likely strike his opposite fore with his hind hooves, creating injury and distress. If you put sport boots on this becomes less risky, but as I stated earlier I do not believe in asking horses to execute in any way that will cause them pain. What I do recommend is that you slow your horse to a slow walk to first learn these movements, only increasing his energy as he becomes adept at them. Further you should understand that if your gaited horse is most comfortable moving in a racking gait or a stepping pace his topline will likely be held in a more difficult posture to easily manage many of the bending exercises commonly required for the leg yield maneuvers. This is just one more reason to keep your gaited horse to the walking gait with the released and fluid topline that it promotes.

Another thing I would ask you to consider is that many dressage instructors who do not have extensive experience with gaited horses and may encourage a quiet, yet firmly constant contact with and through the bit. If you have a racking, trotting or pacing horse this particular practice becomes less problematic, but for those horses that flatfoot walk, running walk or foxtrot this firm yet constant bit contact (even if quiet) will frequently cause the horse to increase the essential tension of his topline in response. This tension may eventually alter his gait and push him away from center toward that pace, trot or rack. A traditional dressage instructor with little understanding of gait bio-mechanics may promote instruction that inhibits the natural and needed head movement that your horse should have.

What I advocate and practice is learning to connect through the bit with a connection that is never maintained with constant contact but rather through light intermittent touches and releases that both reward and free your horse for self carriage and balance. As previously described I recommend a rein hold with thumb and forefinger while using the remaining

three fingers of each hand to collect the rein for contact or release the rein for freedom of movement.

I strongly encourage you to work at dressage exercises, listen to all the great advice and coaching from your dressage instructor but understand these needs of your horse to maintain gait and give him the release and lightness to carry that gait. Connection through release is the best way to communicate while encouraging your horse to listen closely to light rein touches. Connection outside of constant contact is not "throwing away" your communication at all, but rather enhances it to another level. I am releasing my horse into gait and I assert that true dressage masters would understand, respect and encourage this.

LIFTING THE SHOULDERS

The positioning and carriage of the head and neck are intricately involved in how a horse is able to move and use his shoulders, as well as his front-to-back balance. In this manner it directly *AFFECTS HIS GAIT AND THE QUALITY OF THAT GAIT*. When studying the skeletal structure of a horse from the shoulders forward we can see how his neck positioning and carriage has direct *AUTHORITY* over how he is able to use his shoulders. When a horse telescopes the cervical vertebrae forward (and down) this action helps lift the base of cervical arch to release his shoulders into a loose and reaching stride. Just as important, lifting the lower neck enables him to lighten his frontend at the same time he engages the power of his backend. Conversely, when he lifts his head as he would when bracing against or evading a bit he contracts the musculature along the topline which shortens as it contracts and does not allow this telescoping movement. As the cervical vertebrae become jammed by this shortening of the neck his shoulders will most often become locked and braced in a dropped or sunken attitude. These braced horses tend

to suspend in their weight transfer, jogging with their front legs rather than rolling and reaching; using more elbow, knee and fetlock push rather than reaching forward through the shoulder. The sunken attitude also promotes a heavy on the fore balance that will contribute to hollowness and stumbling.

There is a natural "S" shaped curvature in the cervical vertebrae when the neck is relaxed. Beneath the bottom downward curve of the "S" there are hammock-like muscles that enable the horse to lift this area when they contract and shorten. Both the longus colli and the scalenus muscles are what enable a horse to lift his lower neck, sometimes called lifting his withers, as he stretches his neck forward and rounds his poll down. If a rider applies force to the bit while the "S" curve remains in a downward attitude that bit pressure will lock down this curve in that position and actually *INHIBIT* his ability to lift it up with these hammock muscles. The topline trapezius and rhomboideus muscles *MUST RELAX* to allow both the forward stretch as well as the lift from below. It is quite normal for a horse to pull back away from bit pressure which invariably involves contracting this topline muscles. Their bracing engagement works against the need to lengthen the neckline for the base of the neck to lift upward.

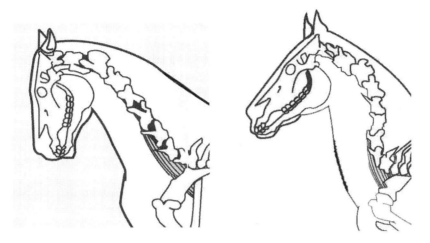

Figure 9.1

Horses ridden consistently with the downward locked attitude of their lower neck will demonstrate visible muscular conformation tendencies with a forward throat bulge frequently called *elk or ewe* neck. This common neckline distortion accompanied by the sunken area in front of the withers and a flat topline forward, are all indications of a horse that is evading behind or bracing against the bit with this lower curve prominently visible in the shape of the neck. If your horse shows these conformation characteristics please invest the time to bit train them to achieve soft and responsive bit engagement. This will not only make gaiting easier and riding more effortless, but will also help rebuild and sculpt a more traditional musculature of the neck.

If you only learn a few things from this book, I truly hope the importance of teaching your horse to lift his lower neck is high on that list. Experienced trainers within disciplines from dressage to reining will tell you that this lift allows any horse to become more athletic and supple; more versatile and mobile because it helps shift his weight back and promotes lightness in the front. Lift of the withers

improves lateral balance and increases the fluid action of this primary movement, as well as helping keep the backend more engaged which is critical for a quality walking gait. To see this demonstrated in a horse at liberty, watch as a stallion approaches a strange horse, be it mare, stud or gelding. When the stallion blooms up at another stallion or when flirting with a mare, you'll see extreme roundness of the cervical arch reaching down to the base of his neckline as his face comes onto more vertical carriage. What this posture does is prepares them to lift their front off the ground whether for fighting or mounting the mare.

To achieve lift as well as enable better reach of the shoulders a horse needs to telescope the vertebrae of the neckline forward almost reaching for the bit. This encourages contraction of the hammock muscles (scalenus and longus colli) below the vertebrae at the base of the neck while at the same time allowing the topline muscles (trapezius and rhomboideus) to release and stretch. Another movement that is extremely important in helping him lift at the lower neck or withers is the flexing of his poll softly and willingly. Let me stress that for consistent self carriage THIS FLEXION MUST BE GIVEN. If you try to force, frame or pull at his mouth to MAKE him flex, the essential tension that results from that force will totally defeat this effort.

I believe it was this desire for lightness and lift of the base of the neck that prompted so many to utilize the inhumane practice of Rollkur. The hyper flexion (over flexion) of the neck is really the only way to force this lift. While these trainers recognize the need to this lift they were evidently ignorant of how the train their horse to give it and resorted to a punishingly harsh framing of the neckline through the bit.

Many gaited riders do not also realize that any attempt by them to force or pull the head upward for any reason also encourages the horse to brace those topline muscles that lock that lower curve of the neck in a downward attitude. We're back to that same *catch 22* we spoke of before where the incorrect action of the rider contributes to the very problem his action is trying to resolve.

The movement of telescoping forward and giving at the poll is what I call LEADING WITH THE EARS. Others have called it *looking through the bridle.* The best way to encourage the release of the topline cervical muscles is to ask him to first lower his head and softly **give** to the bit with voluntary poll flexion that brings his face more on the vertical while lowered. This posture sets the horse up to give you lightness through the base of his neckline. Your goal is to watch for and feel the front of the saddle actually rise slightly as the horse stretches forward with his ears and lifts his lower neck. So if you're having difficulty with the lower neck lift, I strongly suggest you reread and continue practicing the bit training chapter and get your horse softer in his responses. You, as a rider training your horse need to learn the feel of this and understand its importance.

Backend engagement is critical for powerful walking gaits with real lightness and brilliance of the front end. An experience gaited trainer will tell you that lifting of the shoulders/lower neck not only allows a horse to achieve light locomotion with his frontend, but when coupled with a neutral core significantly encourages and helps maintain engagement of his backend. Whether bracing against or trying to evade the bit, any horse encouraged carrying his head and neck in an elevated posture will find backend engagement to be problematic at best. The very act of engaging those dorsal muscles along the topline of the neck also tends to encourage similar contractions through the entire spine. All of this topline shortening and rigidity tends to encourage lift in the backend at the same time it raises the poll. The topline takes on the rocker shape, sunken in the middle with the extremities lifted.

Don't get me wrong, a horse may learn to raise his head and still preserve the lift at his withers, but this usually takes conditioning and practice to do this while maintaining the proper lightness in front as well as the necessary engagement of the backend. For a majority of horses not yet at that advanced stage of training, backend engagement becomes more difficult the higher his head rises. For far too many the higher the head the more likely they will lower their shoulders, brace and suspend, balancing heavy-on-the-fore and getting light on the backend as counter balance. If a rider, for any reason, causes his horse to raise his head higher than his comfort zone, he will unintentionally encourage the drop of his back into hollow without care and conditioning.

We, as riders and trainers of our horses, can learn to help them alter their head and neck carriage WILLINGLY AND COMFORTABLY, and through that alteration can then directly influence their posture to help achieve the correct and brilliant gait we desire.

SHOULDERS-IN AND LEG YIELDS

My very favorite exercises for encouraging a horse to release through his shoulders and help him stride deep on the backend is the shoulder-in or leg yield, because it not only unlocks their shoulders but encourages the essential lift in the base of the neck. Basically the shoulder-in is a leg yield where the horse is asked to bend around your driving leg with his head lightly to one side moving forward at his shoulder while carrying a three track through his body. A three track is where the inside shoulder will have its own track, the inside hind follows the outside shoulder in a center track and finally the outside hind carries its own track.

Many dressage enthusiasts feel the shoulder-in is the first step for a horse learning to collect, and indeed if you define collection as engaged hindquarters and lightened front end this is what you can expect. I guess the beginning of collection is appropriate, and hindquarter engagement, back strengthening, lifting of the shoulder and yielding to your leg are all solid goals for our gaited horses as well. Because this is an exercise best engaged at a walk, I think over collecting into the trot are less of a risk for our gaited horses.

Before you begin working the shoulder-in with your horse you need to have established the lateral movements away from your leg pressure with the working the corners exercise described back in chapter 8. You should further have the bit training for the vertical nod from chapter 7 well established. This will help your horse avoid throwing his nose out and raising his head as you ask him to move diagonally into a bend by encouraging him to keep his neckline rounded and level as his nose comes in.

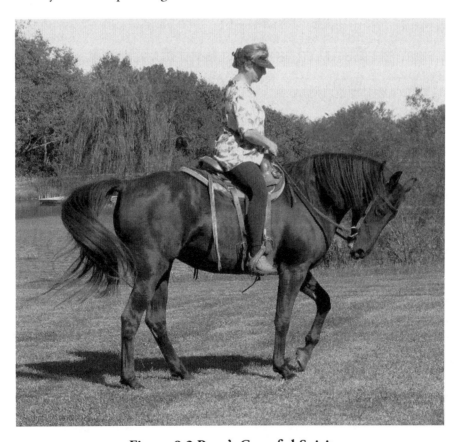

Figure 9.2 Papa's Graceful Spirit

It is important to realize that a shoulder-in can often be a confusing movement for horses that have not yet learned to move in a direction OTHER THAN following their nose. Therefore I recommend starting off by asking for a shoulder nod to one side, repeat a few times to polish his response. Then from that standstill bit movement I then advise adding lateral movement by applying leg pressure (constant and firm), holding and waiting while supporting through the rein. Your horse may not get it at first, so *please be patient.* If you have a riding crop to assist with a light tap on his shoulder just in front of your pressing leg it might help him understand to move laterally away from the leg pressure. For many horses the head bending away from the desired direction will totally confuse them at first.

If your horse really does not understand, many will respond better by learning to move off your leg while walking forward. For these horses you should start walking them slowly in a small, 10 meter circle while applying pressure just behind the girth line with your inside leg and supporting through the rein to keep them bent.

Remember your horse learns from your release, so as soon as you feel those first hesitant steps outward, you need to release all pressure immediately to tell him this is correct. Yea! Reward him and repeat, getting just a step at a time and releasing to reward. Train using the Four R's just like everything else. Eventually you will release and request while your horse takes leading step after leading step. Once you can consistently get a widening circle you are ready to transition this movement down the wall or rail in a straight line. Keep your steps slow and limit to stringing together just a few steps early on. This is a new movement for your horse and you do not want to make him sore in any way. Let him stretch his muscles into it for 2 or 3 strides, release into a straight walk and then bend to the other side. It can take many days to get him accustomed to this movement and we want to keep his attitude positive and interested.

Note: whenever I am training any new movement that involves the head and neck bending or collecting, I always finish by releasing into a stretch to the ground or drop the head low cue to encourage relaxation and stretching out the top line. I also use this when transitioning down from a high energy movement that involves a lot of lift such as the canter. It helps the horse to relax and rewards him for good effort while bringing his energy level down quickly. This stretch to the ground is also a great way to start a very fast and forward horse off for his workout; to kind of start him off right by stretching out, engaging his backend and setting the tempo at slow until you ask him to bring it up.

Part III – NATURAL GAIT CORRECTION

The premise of natural horsemanship is the concept of asking your horse to change his posture and balance, rather than using the three F's of force, frame and fix. I know there will be those people who pick up this book, look at the table of contents then flip right to these chapters on curing the pace and helping the trotting horse. PLEASE STOP, go back and read the chapters on "GIVE", "Bit Training" and "Power Steering". Everything I teach in the following chapters for altering gait *must come from a place of asking rather than forcing, framing and fixing.* It must be asked with the legs and seat before the bit, so the chapter on Power Steering for Your Horse will be essential.

Applying force IN ANY FORM to a horse, particularly through his head and mouth, naturally produces resistance. Any resistance produces tension, and tension alters gait. The very first time you ask a young horse to follow you on a leadline by applying light pressure he will most likely lock up his legs becoming as mobile as a mountain. The very first time you ask him to move his hindquarters over by applying pressure with your hand, he will most likely lean back into your hand pressure. This is not a willful rebellion, but a natural instinctive reaction for horses. You must **teach** them to move away from your pressure, just as you must teach them to give to your seat and leg, to give to the bit with just an ask cue and not through force.

Using old school training methods of forcing mechanical manipulation will produce a distinctly different movement and attitude in a horse; one of stiffness and resistance rather than fluid give and softness. Once you understand the concept it becomes easy to spot this difference when watching horses move. The change of posture and rebalancing needed to alter gait naturally and brilliantly **must come from within the horse, and be given willingly!**

If you're on the same page with me at this point you will agree that to resort to mechanical fixes is simply an unacceptable way to help your horse. Fixes are temporary Band-Aids that are not beneficial for the orthopedic soundness of our horses over the long run. They are uncomfortable and for the most part should not be considered part of REAL horsemanship. So no matter who tells you to alter his hooves, change his shoes or try a more serious bit, ignore this advice because YOU now understand that your horse needs to find his own gaits from within.

I much prefer training barefoot horses and work with the raw material, so to speak. I'm not opposed to shoeing for soundness when it's time to venture out to the trails, but I recommend most basic training to happen at home on safe ground for two reasons. The first being so you may work with the horse's mind and not have the distractions found on the trail. The second is being able to do this homework with bare hooves which is completely sufficient for most horses without hoof problems and it takes the mechanical influence completely out of the equation. You know that if your horse can carry his gait barefoot he can gait in any shoes you may need him to wear for soundness.

I will focus in this section on the most common off-gait problems routinely encountered throughout many of the gaited breeds, the pace and the trot, because these represent the extreme two beat gaits that commonly plague gaited horse riders, and which are least desirable for a gaited horse. If it's not two beat, most pleasure riders are probably content riding their horse and are probably not spending a great deal of time trying to fine tune the easy gait they're already achieving. Part IV of this book, however, does address just such fine-tune training for the Naturally Brilliant Walking Horse, and provides more helpful details for those pleasure riders who seek to improve the gaits of their horse for the pleasure of working toward a defined goal or from the desire to eventually enter the show or exhibition arenas. Both venues request more of a text book walking horse gait.

By now you have a better understanding of the biomechanics of gait, the abilities and possibilities of your riding partner, and you

are ready to proceed. We progress on to the realm of how we get from point A to point B; how to actually ask our horse to change an off-gait into the smooth pleasurable gait we want and that will be comfortable for him to carry with effortless balance and self carriage.

DEVELOPING YOUR PLAN

The first item on our agenda is to evaluate. You must have an understanding about what is causing your horse to be off gait. Remember one of our primary responsibilities in this partnership with our horse is to know what we want. From that informed standpoint we can set small goals that will eventually lead to more involved and complex maneuvers and carriage. We must always start any journey with a first step.

Almost any type of gait correction will depend upon softness and responsiveness from your horse to both your hands through the bit as well as to your seat and leg cues. Achieving this responsiveness comes through the bit training, working the corners, adding the power steering as well as the shoulders-in while continuing to get lighter and lighter with those cues. With those tools we can start working to answer these primary questions:

- Can we ask our horse to carry his head where we need him to? His head and neck carriage is a HUGE tool for helping a horse change his core posture.
- Do we have control or direct influence of both his speed and cadence? Teaching him to rate his gait tempo to your seat and legs allows you to slow down and control his upward transitions from the foundation of the flatfoot walk, gradually increasing his energy while pushing the envelope of isochronal walking cadence for increased speed.
- Can we feel his balance? Understanding how your horse is balancing front to back

at the flatfoot walk, and how that balance changes as he increases his speed will give tremendous insight for needed corrections to that carriage. Feeling at what point he disengages his backend and loses his controlled impulsion tells you exactly where and when you should help briefly support his upward transitions.

Picturing the easy gaits on a linear graph, you would see that those gaits of most even timing are directly in the middle. While a graph like this helps people understand the relation of the easy gaits to each other as well as the two beat extremes as a dimension of timing, I like to picture them as more like an archer's target, with the most isochronal gaits being dead center bull's-eye. When shooting for a target most of us will aim for the middle and be happy the closer we can get to that middle. When training a pleasure horse I always set my goal for dead-center even timing as I train and if the horse finds it a little more comfortable to be slightly lateral or slightly diagonal, I still will have helped him find a four beat gait that is both smooth to ride and easy for him to carry based on his own conformation and abilities. For many horses this is where we will leave it and consider gait correction to be successful for both partners. For those folks who are interested in exhibiting their gaited horses they may desire a little more textbook gait for the exhibition arena and there are many things that can be done to refine these gaits with patience and persistence. But all change must come from

a position of knowledge and understanding
so you're not simply shooting in the dark and
hoping.

Chapter 10 - Curing the Pace

NOTE: IF YOU HAVE NOT YET READ CHAPTERS ON "GIVE", "BIT TRAINING" AND "POWER STEERING" PLEASE DO SO BEFORE PROCEEDING.

Though most of you may have identified the problem, identifying the cause comes next. "Why does my horse always pace?" is one of the primary questions that I am asked by gaited horse owners. I hear this just slightly more than "what do I do with this trotting horse?" So let's open this discussion with the many reasons that could be causing your horse to default to a hard riding, 2 beat pace.

1. Immaturity so that a horse's back cannot support a rider without sinking into a hollow frame supported by the dorsal muscling.
2. Poor saddle fit, or a saddle placed improperly causing his back to drop away from stress or brace against that discomfort.

SOLVE THE PHYSICAL FIRST!

Deal with those issues that you can easily solve right away. Of the list above many of these are issues that can be easily resolved with a little effort and understanding on the part of the rider.

AGE: I am opposed to working two year old horses under saddle - period. I do not recommend working three year old horses for anything except careful and deliberate schooling in an arena situation where the

3. Bit evasion causing him to lift or toss his head high, engaging dorsal muscles. Causes:
   a. Teeth issues
   b. Bad bit or bit positioning
   c. Harsh hands of the rider
   d. Lack of training for bit acceptance
4. Downhill balance or build (often a result of immaturity) as well as head carriage.
5. Naturally high strung worrier temperament causing the above posture.
6. Performance horse bred as a hard wired pacer. This actually occurs less that you might think.

I've talked about the importance of the horse's comfort and how we should always address the physical needs of our horse before we begin serious training.

ENVIRONMENT AND FOOTING ARE CONTROLLED. Young horses are at a tremendous disadvantage in trying to carry the load of an adult rider with their immature bodies. While they may be able to carry a person from point A to point B, maneuvering an obstacle, climbing hills, and pushing for any kind of real speed is simply unreasonable and even hazardous for them. Because their joints are not only softer with active growth plates, their tendons are more elastic and their muscles are simply weaker. All of these combine to create a situation *WHERE ALL IT TAKES IS A STUMBLE*, a misplaced hoof slipping out from under them, or an awkward catch when backing up and suddenly they've strained a joint, ligament, tendon to the point where it must heal. This healing process often creates scar tissue as most healing processes do. The nature of scar tissue is to be sturdier than the original tissue, but less elastic. The resulting lack of elasticity often results in unbalanced gait or shortened and off strides. Scar tissue often compromises the range of motion in that joint for the rest of that horse's life. These injuries will also increase the likelihood of arthritis later as the horse ages and reduce the life of his usefulness. The unfortunate truth is that for many horses their usefulness will dictate their life span and the quality of that life. Tremendous care should always be taken to maintain good orthopedic posture and attitudes for increased longevity.

I hope everyone will treat their young horse is like a bottle of fine wine, and be willing to invest the time to allow them to mature so they (and you) can realize their full potential.

BITTING AND SADDLE FIT: Please read chapter 3's section on both saddle fit and bitting to understand how this unrelenting discomfort will cause your horse to brace, hollow and throw his head up. A horse's natural reaction to discomfort is to try to brace their body and avoid any movement that makes it worse. I am often reminding people to imagine wearing a horribly uncomfortable pair of shoes and how miserable it would be to even stand around in them, let alone do much walking. We should not expect our horses to relax and go neutral through their topline if we're placing our weight onto a saddle that is an uncomfortably poor fit.

BIT AVOIDANCE MAY BE MORE THAN FIT. Be honest in evaluating how you ride. Do you frequently find yourself maintaining contact on the bit for no particular reason or purpose? Have you been told that a gaited horse must have pressure in his mouth to perform gait? Do you often feel wobbly, top heavy and unstable sitting on your horse? Give yourself a break and understand that most of us have been taught wrong in our early exposures to gaited horses (really all horses). Just look at the bits we were told to use on these horses. Can we be blamed for accepting the advice of the very people who sold us the horse?

I'm going to be honest with you. If you simply want to be a twice a month hobby rider, then do yourself a favor and buy a horse that's already been trained; a been there, done that kind of horse that will be worry and hassle free for you. While it may cost you a little more, if you're not prepared to become part of the training equation and fully expect to ride this horse as he is, you could end up paying more in other ways. Be realistic and honest with yourself. Both you and the horse you choose will be better for that honest evaluation.

If, however, you enjoy and embrace the challenge of communicating with your horse; if you feel passionate about being an equestrian and want a horse that is a partner and friend in adventure then you are mentally prepared to invest your time in becoming a better partner for your horse. That means learning to balance better, to ride with less hand support, to use a leg and seat method of communicating that is kinder and more consistent for him.

Once you have made that commitment you should be ready to work with your horse on his bit training. I firmly feel *THAT BIT TRAINING IS AN INVESTMENT IN YOUR HORSE*, but it's more than that. It's an investment in your partnership and in yourself because riding your horse is a part of who you are. Learning to ride with kinder, less intrusive bit communication will not only benefit your current horse, but will help you with any horse you may ride in the future and become more stable in the saddle today.

CONDITIONING THE TOP LINE

Now comes the harder issues; those physical problems that need to be overcome to better allow your horse to lose his ingrained pacing habit.

There are horses that are heavy on the fore, and there are horses that are built downhill, and not always are they one in the same. Those built downhill means the crest of their withers is slightly lower than the sacrum above their hips (more specifically the base of the neck alignment is lower than the core of the loins, but this alignment is more difficult for the layman to see). Downhill build is not at all uncommon in gaited horses, though many believe it should be. The blame rests with breeders being more concerned about bloodlines, color genetics, and monster backend stride as priorities over solid conformation and athletic balance. Breeder concerns often side more toward what makes horses marketable to the buying public or what will win in the performance arenas.

For some endeavors a downhill horse is not a handicap. For those activities that revolve around speed or racing events a slightly downhill build may actually assist the horse rather than hinder. However for our purposes as a saddle horse a downhill build makes the job of balancing a rider an uphill battle... forgive me, I just couldn't resist. The conformationally downhill horse is at a disadvantage in trying to lift his lower neck and lighten his front in relation to his hind quarters. This disadvantage is not helped at all by any mechanical effort of the rider to force the horse to rebalance. Rebalancing and lifting the fore is a process of conditioning the topline and core muscles while strengthen the haunches to enable the desired shift of balance.

Achieving a neutral topline and working a default isochronal walk with proper backend engaged will set a horse up for a successful intermediate gait without sliding off toward lateral pairing. Getting the poll lower than his withers, teaching him to soften to the bit and give at the poll all help him achieve the evenly timed walking gait. I recommend treating the walk as home base and always returning to this foundation four beat gait after every transition whether or not that transition is successful. The trail walk and the flatfoot walk should be trained as his default gears where he can always be comfortable and rewarded with a release of all bit contact from a relaxed and balanced rider. It is in this even four beat gait that he releases most if not all of his core tension and works all the muscles of that core in fluid synchronicity.

To accomplish this we need our horse to condition himself to avoid bracing the topline. He must learn to bear the weight of the rider with this released topline. Depending upon his conformation and balance may possibly take several weeks or even months for him to accomplish. Start with the trail walk as his default gait and as he progresses in his training the flatfoot walk will become his new default gait. You can NEVER overwork the flatfoot walk so always come back to this.

ALTERING THE CORE: If you think about the spine of a horse as being like the limb of an archer's bow where the muscles of his core act upon this bow like a string to bend it one direction or another, then it becomes more clear how to ask the horse to use his muscles to change his posture and balance. First off, understand that muscles only contract (shorten) and release (lengthen). Muscles never push. To wave your arm back and forth requires the muscles on either side to contract while the opposite side releases. Therefore to round up the topline we will need the muscles below the spine (the abdominal/ ventral muscles) to contract while those above the spine (dorsal muscles) release. Keep in mind that our goal is really not to seriously change vertebral alignment so much as to alter the muscle contractions and bracing. It is the muscle contractions that actually change the gait being carried not the alignment of vertebrae.

The change of posture is not always easy for horses that have traveled with a braced topline for many years. These horses have very strong and over developed dorsal muscling and under developed, weaker ventral (abdominal) muscles. My rule of thumb is that for each YEAR a horse has been allowed to carry a rider incorrectly, you should expect it to take a MONTH of consistent and patient riding to correct. So if you have a ten year old gelding that was started at three and has been allowed to carry a dominant pace for seven years, you must generally expect it to take around seven months for him to overcome the muscles he's built and to develop and use new muscles. Of course there are variables that directly affect this calculation by how often he's been ridden in his incorrect carriage and how often you are now riding and asking him to correct. This does not mean it will take seven months to teach him to carry a smooth gait, just that he may continue to try defaulting toward the off-gait for that long. His new muscles will need those months to become dominant and for him to become more set in his new gait.

Three primary cues, or pressures can be used to help horses learn to round up and to alter their muscles usage.

1. The head needs to lower where **the poll is below the withers**. This does a number of things but primarily as the head lowers it applies pressure on the dorsal muscles to encourage release and helps 'pull out the hollow'. Lowering his head also encourages the horse to relax which further promotes a natural release of the topline muscles. I highly recommend employing a drop the head cue from chapter 7 to train your horse to carry and keep his head low while moving forward in gait. You should further support this posture by keeping your own hands low with the reins, applying any light touches on the bit in a backward motion rather than upward. Pull lightly toward your knees or thighs rather than toward your waist or chest.

2. The backend needs to drop into engagement. You will note that I talk about backend engagement in a number of the training sections, but especially about contributing to a quality walking gait. The horse needs to release his hips into a rolling, reaching stride rather than carry a braced, locked or jogging backend. Bending through leg yields, lateral movements, and slowing his overall speed will all encourage him to maintain a sweeping striding backend. The rider really needs to focus and learn what backend engagement feels like, otherwise you're shooting in the dark for a target you only vaguely know is there. The engaged backend will have more front-to-back push on your hips as they mirror his hips. Also the deeper and longer he strides the bigger this front-to-back push becomes. Next time you ride, find a safe arena or paddock area that you feel secure in and while sitting tall and balanced, close your eyes and feel the sweep of each stride in the horse's backend. Your hips will move forward as each of his legs lifts to sweep forward for planting. Speed the horse up and then feel how the movement in your hips alters and you will begin to understand how vital this knowledge is. You will have difficulty in training your horse to remain in any gait that you cannot feel.

3. The base of the neck or withers needs to lift. You may recall that I talk about this particular movement at length in the **chapter on bit training**. This lifting *IS* what a horse does when he rebalances

and lightens his front. It also goes hand in hand with backend engagement. You can encourage this action by lowering the head, asking for vertical flexion, dropping the backend into engagement and using your calves at the girth line to apply a lifting aid with your legs to help encourage this. With the backend and the head/neck dropped the final ingredient of a round topline is the lift in the middle. Help him understand and accomplish this by giving you poll flexion and vertical face while his neckline is level with his withers. First down, then round. Please take care that you never force or frame this position. You need to coax him to lift his withers and applying force is completely counterproductive to your goals.

A word of caution here; don't be surprised if, as your horse begins to release his topline and alter his balance and posture, you begin to see a *DRAMATIC CHANGE IN HIS GAIT AND TIMING*. After all that is our goal. However many people may be concerned when a here-to-fore confirmed pacer suddenly releases, rounds *AND SWITCHES ALL THE WAY TO A TROT*. This is not at all uncommon, particularly as the horse is bending through curves while at gait and should never be considered a bad thing. It is both a part of his evolution and a moment of enlightenment for you that you have a horse that can not only trot but may actually prefer to trot when you take away the physical reasons for his dorsal dominant topline that was causing his pace. I see this evolution all the time and I celebrate these moments because it not only tells me that the horse is connecting to his conformationally supported gait, but he's learning that he can change. You've opened up his repertoire of gait and introduced him to the wide range of variations he has available to him. From here it is a learning process for you both on exactly how to fine tune his gait to the middle away

from the extremes he has now shown himself capable of. You know if he paces and he can trot then he is fully capable of all those gaits in between.

My personal preference is to allow a horse to find his trot and actually use it for several days. These are new muscles he needs to develop and have at his disposal, so don't freak out and yank his head up trying to shy away from a new gear. Using the trot as a building and condition tool is advisable and provides some short cut to getting a pacer to be set to a new isochronal default gait.

I've honestly heard some gaited horses owners express such uninformed concern that any horse that trots would be shot; they will not have it on their farm! Well, I'm sorry to tell these folks that the overwhelming majority of gaited horses in their pastures have this gear readily available if they only knew it. But their antiquated riding practices of force frame and fix make it highly unlikely that they will find this gait while carrying them in the saddle, and if asked they are probably happy about this because they would not know what to do with a gaited horse that trots. If you understand the biomechanics of why your horse has altered to the trot, you realize the solution is right there in front of you. If lowering his head and rounding his topline helped him find a more diagonal timing, does it not make sense that a more level, neutral or even hollow core will push him right back toward the lateral side? Your goal is to shoot for the middle of a neutral released core where he will effortlessly engage in evenly timed gaits that are smooth and pleasurable for you both. If, in the unlikely event you find your horse so solidly confirmed to the trot (possible but not probable) after learning to release the hollow core, then go to the chapter in this book dealing with Helping the Trotting Horse and learn how your horse can learn to become less confirmed in that gear.

In the illustration here you see the same

horse being ridden in the same tack on the same day. In the first I'm allowing this horse to default to his pace because he is still at the beginning of his training. In the second I've asked him to lower his head and find his walking gait.

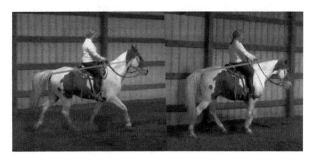

Figure 10.1 Luke

There are two things I'd like you to note about his carriage. First is when pacing his head is high and he seems almost to sink at the base of his neck, showing how he is balanced to the front and seems to almost lift his sacrum in response to the tense dorsal muscles he's carrying. Now compare that to the photo where I have him more released. His topline is more level, his head is lower and his backend is solidly engaged and striding quite nicely. I've drawn a line in both photos from the tail dock across the pummel of the saddle to illustrate the topline change. Also note how the saddle has leveled up as he lowers his head rather than tilting down in the pacing photo.

The second thing I'd like to point out is how his timing has become more even or isochronal. Both photos show this horse at point of weight transfer on the backend and during even (isochronal) timing the front *should be* exactly midstride. While he's not completely even in the second photo he is obviously more so, with his front, weight bearing leg is closer to midstride.

EXERCISES FOR BALANCE

I want to focus specifically on balance and detail those exercises that will improve a horse's self carriage and balance. While these exercises are wonderful for any horse they all are wonderful tools for getting the dorsal dominant pacer to release and rebalance his core. The relaxed core is so vital for both gait and orthopedic soundness that I felt it deserved this recap.

- Drop the head cue will help to pull the hollow from the core topline of the thoracolumbar arch as well as encourage the horse to keep his backend engaged in the walking gaits. This also opens the door for the horse to lift the base of his neck/wither area for improved lightness on the fore and better hind impulsion.

- Cavaletti or walk overs encourage the horse to drop his head and round his topline as he picks his way over. Do not try to rush this exercise. It is not a speed event, and is more beneficial to start slowly so the horse may focus on the obstacle. As your horse learns to walkover obstacles without banging, bumping or clunking them you may encourage him to increase his speed. This will tell you a great deal about his awareness of his feet and his athletic ability to adapt.

- Shoulder-in's and leg yields are where the shoulders are bent slightly away from his direction of travel as the horse yields to a driving inside leg of the rider. A slight pull on one rein encouraging the head toward the one o'clock at the right or the eleven o'clock at the left while the horse continues forward on a three-track bend, with the inside hind leg tracking on its own, while the other hind tracks behind the diagonal opposite fore and the outside fore tracks on its own. These bending exercises will encourage release at the shoulder, lift of the lower neck and help the backend re-engage at a striding deep walk.

REIN-BACK DONE RIGHT

The reinback is simply a back up asked for by the rider executed with a lowered head and engaged core. Because of both the posture and the engagement required to execute, and because it can be utilized at a very slow and deliberate speed to start, the rein-back becomes one of the best exercises for helping a horse improve all of these.

A horse should be asked for each deliberate step of his backup from a posture of lowered head, rounded core and coiled loins. From a stopped position you first ask him to drop his head with a give at the poll for a very round and low neckline. *FROM THIS POSTURE* you sit back slightly, bringing your legs forward, alternately squeeze and release as he accomplishes each step. If your horse throws his head up in resistance you must ask him to lower it again before proceeding with the rein-back. To be of maximum benefit this exercise needs roundness of the entire topline and it is particularly important he keep his loins coiled at the sacrum. If you are not certain your horse is not working correctly, have someone watch his hooves closely. When the posture is correct, his hooves should lift and place in

- As you ride, your seat should move with the horse. To encourage lift and lightness in the front that will combat both hollow heavy on the fore as well as foxtrot heavy on the fore, hug at the girth line with a lifting motion of your calves, while you cue for a drop the head round and down with your reins. This should be a singular motion followed by a quick release that should help your horse to avoid falling onto his fore and/or encourage him to rebalance toward the rear.

a closely diagonal pairing; a foxtrot timing if you like.

If a horse resists backing, lifts his head, pulls the dorsal muscles to dominant or uncoils his loins he, in effect, disconnects his backend from his front. When this happens the backup becomes difficult and possibly even uncomfortable. He may try to step back with his fore but his hindquarters feel like their stuck. If or when you finally do manage to get backward movement, it is disjointed and unaligned with the hindquarters trying to swing to the side and get out of the way of his front. The steps lose their diagonal timing as well. Everything about the maneuver becomes a struggle for the horse and downright ugly to watch. Stop. Get the posture correct first. Only when your horse is in proper posture can he give you correct, effortless movement. Start slowly as mentioned and only ask for faster movement as his balance and coordination support it. I recommend making the rein-back part of your daily exercises for all the important muscle development and coordination it promotes.

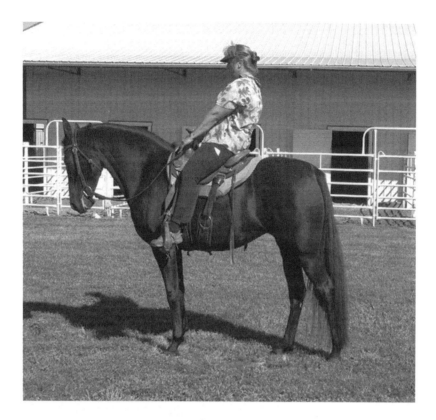

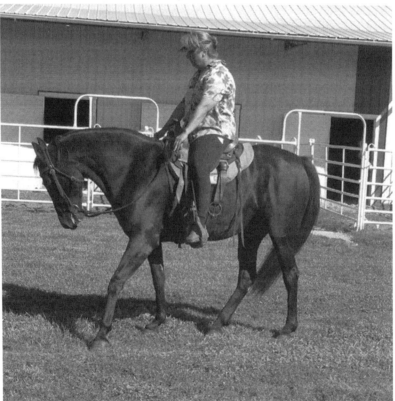

Figure 10.2 Papa's Graceful Spirit

Chapter 11 - Helping the Trotting Horse

NOTE: IF YOU HAVE NOT YET READ CHAPTERS ON "GIVE", "BIT TRAINING" AND "POWER STEERING" PLEASE DO SO BEFORE PROCEEDING.

The gaited horse that moves toward a default trot is not a problem to work with as many may have you believe. He is most often simply rounding a little too much through his core by engaging his ventrum. He may also show a tendency to go heavy on the fore leading him to trot from the backend forward.

I want to insist that the default trotting gaited horses are tremendously gaited despite what many believe. It is my experience that they actually settle into an easy gait more firmly than most default pacing horses. So never feel like a trotting gaited horse is any less valuable. Many are greatly desired because of their natural abilities for athletic maneuvers as well as readily picking up the canter, and often being more sure-footed than a pacing horse. For these reasons and more they make excellent pleasure horses, as well as versatile working horses.

From the isochronal walking gait a default trotter may stretch his nose forward and sometimes even down, shifting his balance forward. Hindquarters that were previously engaged at a walking gait will tend to get behind and uncoil somewhat as his speed outstrips his comfortable walking reach. He compensates this by disengaging his backend into a jogging step just a half beat before

his fore likewise tightens and pairs into a fully diagonal trot. His diagonal timing is supported by the rounding through the core with what I call ventral dominance while his sacrum allows the hips to brace and begin jogging in a suspended weight transfer.

It is important to note this inclination to transition into a trot backend first. At this point most gaited horses will be at or close to a foxtrot, but also just a heartbeat away from a solid two beat jog trot. It is often a transition phase that does not last more than a step or two so if you're asleep at the wheel you'll miss it and suddenly find your horse trotting along.

It is significant to understand that the trot is a more energy expensive gait. It costs the horse more energy as compared to the walking gaits because it requires more upward loft of both the horse and the rider's weight. He transitions to this trot anticipating that he will be asked for greater speed than his walk can support. While the rounded core is stronger to support a rider, it is also less comfortable to the horse because the very same impact we experience in the saddle is being likewise felt by our horse upon his back as our weight thumps down. Because the trot uses more energy and is less comfortable for the horse it is usually not too difficult to persuade him with a little patient effort to maintain and extend the smooth and comfortable four beat walking gaits. The discomfort and energy cost of trotting with a rider gives him strong incentive to stay in gait. This is why I recommend NOT posting when your horse moves into a trot. Let your weight settle into the saddle with every thump while you're asking him to correct back to the softer four beat. Take advantage of this natural incentive to gait.

There are three basic maneuvers that I want you to teach your horse to be used as tools to break up his evolution from walking gait to a trot.

- Flexing and giving to the bit at the poll, willingly bringing his nose in toward his chest in a vertical give, allows us to counter his inclination to both stretch his nose out to balance forward.
- Giving softly to the bit with the bend, progressing to a shoulder-in or leg yield will allow you to bend his core slightly while maintaining a more or less forward energy flow.
- Lowering AND lifting his head and neck posture also helps keep him in balance for an engaged walking backend.

These are your tools to help him resist his natural inclination to transition into the trot. Before you begin active gait correction, practice these maneuvers to get a consistent and soft responsiveness from a stopped position. Difficulty with these at a stop means they will be twice as difficult once his feet are moving. Here is one more place that your prior preparation will pay off. Invest the time to get the desired results. Further, if after you are well into gait correction mode he becomes stiff and resistant again, stop and refresh these tools.

As I outline above, a horse will typically move to the trot slightly backend first, so we must be vigilant to watch for the first signal of his intension to transition his hindquarters. Most horses will give us clues to their intention to change gait if we pay close attention. Often they will stretch their nose out, sometimes

lowering their head as well and gather their core with a little more roundness, then finally lightening the backend first. This process may vary a little from horse to horse and your job is to evaluate *AND KNOW YOUR HORSE* and how he makes his transition.

Evaluating and learning the feel of this will be easier if you can slow down your horse's transition by asking him to very *GRADUALLY* increase his energy level from the walking gait. Don't kick 'em up quickly because an abrupt cue will always be interpreted by your horse that you want a different gait and that's what he'll try to give you. You simply want him to extend the walking gait in both speed and tempo. So be subtle in how you ask him to increase his energy output, remaining balanced and quiet in the saddle. Sometimes all it takes is draping your legs back toward the back position without actually applying pressure. Sometimes a simple leaning forward a little in the saddle will likewise encourage an increase in speed. However your horse best responds your goal is make this ask for energy to be slow, and deliberate.

As you feel (and learn) your horse is reaching the top end of his walking speed be ready for his initial alteration and transition.

- If he reaches his nose out and down, counter by using the above tools to ask him to bring his nose back in, his poll and neck up at level with or slightly higher than his withers.
- If he gets a lot of tension through his topline with excessive collection and rounding in his core, use the one rein half-halt much like a mini-bend with a leg yield to break up his rounded core with bend and get him to relax it again. Bend and release first to one side – pause - then to the other. Never holding the bend for more than a second or two.
- IF you feel him begin to tighten his hips, preparing to jog, use your weight in the

saddle with *A SOFT SIDE-TO-SIDE SHIFT* as you apply a quick half-halt to check him. The side to side motion is what a pacing or laterally timed gait will feel like, and we want to emulate that motion to encourage him to swing through his hips a little more and help avoid the braced and upward loft of the jog.

ABOVE ALL YOU DO NOT LET HIM TROT. If the above fails then slow your horse, bring him back to the walking speed of his default gait and start again. He will most likely not get it the first time, but your patience and persistence can start his learning process. Many of these trotters will experience an epiphany moment somewhere around two to three weeks into training where the light bulb of comprehension suddenly turns on and glows brightly. They have an "ah hah!" moment when they understand what you're asking and will begin giving it to you to the best of their ability. For the trotting horse this is a huge milestone that changes their training from "what do you want?" to "I can do that, but only so fast so far". From there it is conditioning and training their muscles to extend their walking gaits while remaining light on their front end and driving with engagement on their backend.

Most trotters will find a faster walking gait to be more pleasurable and easier on them than the trot ever was. This helps to cement this gait into their muscle memory quickly and quite permanently. Unlike the pacer who may have a tendency to regress after several weeks or months of no riding, the trotter becomes quite set in his gaits once he overcomes his trot tendencies. These horses frequently become so set in gait they are novice-proof with their gait and you can put anyone on them for a successful ride. I'm not saying pacers cannot become as set, but they do tend to take a little more effort and time to get there.

A default trotter will, because of their natural rounding of the core, invariably find a quality three beat canter much easier and more effortless. There are so many facets of the quality canter that are supported by a diagonal timing and rounded frame that this is a real bonus for those who own default-to-trot gaited horses. Don't be intimidated if your horse defaults in this direction. It will take a little more effort to correct initially but these horses are every bit as gaited as any hard pacer out there. We just need to show them the light and they'll give you the smooth ride you've always dreamed of riding.

Chapter 12 – Canter for the Gaited Horse

NOTE: *IF YOU HAVE NOT YET READ CHAPTERS ON "GIVE", "BIT TRAINING" AND "POWER STEERING" PLEASE DO SO BEFORE PROCEEDING.*

I think most of us have heard the myth that *"you shouldn't canter a gaited horse."* Not! This claim has always seemed so totally strange to me considering that the rocking chair canter is one of the three signature gaits of the Tennessee Walking Horse, and both Walkers and Foxtrotters are not considered to be finished horses until this third gait is in their repertoire. I can only imagine this belief of the inability, OR INADVISABILITY, of cantering your gaited horse came about for two reasons. The overriding factor would be the difficulty of getting a correct and effortless canter from a horse that is moving by default in a more dorsal dominant posture. And possibly because as a horse learns to pick up and carry an easy rolling canter they often learn to prefer that gear over the other intermediate gaits, particularly the racking gaits which are often require a great deal more energy.

I certainly agree that you should establish your intermediate gaits before training and riding a canter, but a slow rolling canter it is not something anyone should miss out on. The second solution is to make certain to train the canter correctly and to be very distinct, clear and unique with your cue for this gait, allowing the horse to better differentiate the canter cue from other gait cues.

I am a firm believer that the canter is as natural to our gaited horses as it is to any non-gaited breed; and I am a fan, simply put. But I will also admit that if your horse is traveling high headed, hollow and heavy-on-the-fore he's not ready to train for the canter until this posture is corrected. I think most of us have witnessed the appalling habit of riders trying to mechanically lift up their horses into a canter by exaggerated pumping on the reins in a manner that seems more conducive to starting a chain saw than for equitation. This offensive habit is usually a product of mistakenly thinking they're going to lift the horse into a brilliant cantering gait. What they're not realizing is that they are dealing with a horse that's out of balance and their attempt to encourage the canter is actually *CONTRIBUTING TO THE PROBLEM*; making it worse instead of better. The posture and balance needs correction first; otherwise you invariably end up with a poorly balanced and stiff pace-gallop.

THE PACE-GALLOP is a term I coined to describe the biggest fault I regularly see in gaited horses attempting to canter. The term pace-gallop came from both the lateral pairing and the fast, leaping four-beat hoof support. It is a high-headed, dorsal dominant, almost-hitch-and-roll movement that is very lateral in timing. It appears fast and flat with barely any lift and it is not uncommon to see the rider frantically pulling on the reins trying to slow down their horse. Besides being so

Furthermore, it seems that most walkers seem to overwhelmingly lean toward either the four beat pace gallop or the collected three beat rocking chair with no aerial phase. It is a small percentage that finds a middle ground of a correct three beat canter with speed extended to the point where the aerial phase returns, but not so much so that the lateral swing alters it to a four-beat fault. This is something that deserves continued study and research. In the mean time I want to stress that the form of the Rocking Chair Canter continues to be collected and correct.

We find a similar occurrence when watching dressage horses execute a pirouette. This is discussed in an article titled ***Comparison of the Temporal Kinematics of the Canter Pirouette and Collected Canter*** (Burns, 1997) authored by Theresa E. Burns and Hilary M. Clayton published in the Equine Veterinary Journal. Burns and Clayton studied eleven horses executing the pirouette via slow and stop motion video and found that all

eleven were placing this driving hind hoof a fraction of a second *before* the lead hoof lifts off, thereby negating the label of a leaping gait for that movement as well.

I believe a similar balancing mechanism is aiding the walking horse in avoiding any impact resulting from an aerial phase to create a smooth, stepping weight transfer much as we see between supporting pairs at the walking gaits. I also feel that the long stride and reach of the walking horse is what enables them to make this hoof-to-hoof weight transfer with the transverse hooves. Coupled with the slower speed and tempo it becomes quite natural for them to loft up while reaching under for greater support. My conclusion is that the Rocking Chair Canter cannot accurately be labeled as a leaping gait, but rather becomes more of a non-suspending, nonsymmetrical stepping gait. The long reach of the walking horse hindquarters allows him to bridge the normal aerial phase and perform a gait that is still correct, elegant and energy efficient.

DEVELOPING THE CANTER

The canter should not be a quickly taught gait because of the strength and conditioning that is required. Some horses will readily pick it up while others will simply tend to pace faster when you ask them to canter. Those pacing horses will take more patience because their balance and posture is so vital to the correct gait, and they must first address the posture issue before being ready to pick up a quality canter.

Step 1 – Set your horse up to succeed by teaching him to carry himself in correct, BALANCED form. You must train your horse to lose the dorsal dominant core commonly seen in the default pacers; to release his braced topline to walk with an even four-beat, relaxed motion. Train him to work this walking gait with a more rounded posture where the poll is level with the withers. This will encourage hindquarter engagement as well as strengthen

haunch and ventral muscles, both of which are vital to a quality canter. Your horse needs to learn to keep his head low and to quickly respond to your drop-the-head cue *at any gear or speed*. It is important that he remain in this correct walking posture as he learns to gradually increase energy and impulsion while comfortably resisting lifting his head as you put a leg on him. Until he can listen and respond to your leg cues without this instinctive worry reaction, he's not ready to start working on the canter.

Recommended exercises to aid your horse in releasing and rounding his core are Cavaletti walk-over polls, lateral bending, stepping into turns, step-by-step rein-backs, shoulder-ins and down and round stretching into the bit. To be of maximum benefit it is important that all of the above should be executed with the head lowered where THE POLL IS LEVEL WITH, OR

By Anita J Howe

LOWER THAN, THE WITHERS.

Step 2 I recommend training the canter using circles. Many people recommend using hills because it naturally encourages the horse to shift his weight backward and lighten on the front. Eventually, however, even the longest of hills must end and many of us live in less hilly areas. A 20 meter circle or a round pen not only provides a similar effect of encouraging the lightness on the front to negotiate the curve, but also assists us by discouraging the horse's instinct to blast off into a speed gait (pace) losing both form and balance. The added bend through the core also works to discourage hollowness, and helps the horse pick up a correct lead.

Step 3 – Train yourself *NOT* to pull on the horse's head in any upward manner. This instinct to pull upward while asking for canter seems to be almost subconscious for many riders and *YOU REALLY NEED TO LOSE IT.* You must learn to ride with balance, using an independent seat where your primary communication with your horse comes from seat and legs, not from your hands through the reins. Every effort should be made to preserve those reins for much more subtle and delicate communications. Your horse will relax and he will actually listen closer to those rein cues the quieter you are able to keep your hands. Conversely someone who is overpowering with their hands causes a horse to shut down; to brace against and/or evade the bit. These riders become like the proverbial screaming kid that you just want to plug your ears and get away from. Your horse will try to mentally shut you out rather than listen.

To avoid this common pitfall, I recommend if at all possible for riders first to canter on trained horses, learning to do so with no hand support. Until a rider can manage this, he or she is at a disadvantage in trying to train a canter on a novice horse. If you simply do not have any opportunity to learn from an experienced horse, I beg you to be aware of your hands

and keep them soft and quiet on the reins. Out of everything you need to do to train and cue for the canter, comparatively little should involve your hands. A light, fingertip half-halt should be angled *BACKWARD* toward your thighs to block forward run-away movement. It should NEVER be pulled upward toward your shoulders in attempt to lift the horse. Its purpose is not to lift but to lightly capture his forward energy and encourage him to lift himself or rebalance. Remember to cue, not lift; to ask, not force. Your elbows should be *FIXED* by your side with your forearms angled straight toward the bit. *YOUR ELBOWS SHOULD STAY THERE AND NOT MOVE AS YOU CANTER.* Resist any need to move even your wrists most of the time and try keeping everything with the reins isolated to just a fingertip movement.

Step 4 – Learn to ride the cantering hitch-and-roll. Learn to encourage correct movement in your horse by moving **with** the horse. This movement will tell him what you want. When we resist, or counter his natural motion, or block him in any way, we are telling the horse that we don't like or want what he's doing.

To properly ride and encourage your horse for a canter you need to learn precisely *WHEN* and how to ask for it, to apply a light nudge with your calf, to use a very light fingertip half-halt, to rock back with a hip rolling motion that moves with the horse's natural rhythms while giving a light lifting motion with your calves. Learn *when* to roll back on your seat bones, tilting your pelvis, opening up and slightly lifting your knees to allow and encourage him to lift his shoulders. Learn also when to lean forward and repeat the sequence of the cue: the lift, the rollback, the knees.

This motion of moving with your horse is every bit as vital to communicate to him what you want as is the initial cue. Like our movement with our horse to encourage his walking gaits and speed transitions, we use our seat to either be a passive seat because we like his speed, a driving seat to increase his

114

speed, or a resisting seat to slow his tempo.

There is also a consideration of how to sit the canter. Some horses need the constant driving seat to keep them from dropping out. Those horses I ride with the full three-point seat I've described above. Others are more polished and willing and do not require the constant urging from the rider or the repetitive rebalancing of the half-halt. These more polished horses I use a standing or two-point seat that allows the maximum amount of freedom for the horse to execute his gait. The more collected and lofting a rocking chair canter becomes the easier it is for us to sit with a two-point seat allowing greater motion of the horse beneath us.

I further reward a horse for his correct gait by keeping all bit connections to a minimum; particularly as he lifts up. The better he lifts and rolls the lighter I make bit connection. I want to make the up his point of *complete release*, and only making minimal contact at the down point to resist, increase or passively ride his tempo. I want him to enjoy the gait as he learns to go with me, and I do this by removing all pressure when he's moving correctly. Ride with the movement but remove all pressure and cues until you feel him starting to fall out or you need him to change or correct.

Step 5 – Timing is everything! I mentioned above how the savvy rider should *time* their cue as the driving leg is planting. Here are the nuts and bolts about why and how you learn to do this. Many riders are unaware of exactly when the horse's hind legs are planting. So "how" you ask, "can I know when to cue at the proper moment?"

First understand the biomechanics of the isochronal walking gait and its sequences. The hind leg should always be a *half step* ahead of its laterally paired fore leg. When the left hind lifts and swings forward to the mid-point of its stride (the hoof is directly below the hip), is when the left fore is just leaving the ground.

Consequently, as that left fore reaches *its* mid stride, the left hind should be at or near its point of placement. *That* is the moment to cue the right lead canter so the horse is most clear in their understanding of what you want. That moment of left hind plant comes just as the left fore is lifted beneath the point of the shoulder (non weight bearing) and the right fore is under the shoulder, completely weight bearing.

HINT: from the saddle I find it easier to watch the outside shoulder as I prepare to cue a canter. It takes some practice to learn to cue at a specific moment in the stride, so when first learning I suggest following the rhythm of the walking gait in your head while chanting "now, now, now" each time you see that outside shoulder reach its midpoint. This will imprint the rhythm in your head making it easier hit the beat with your cue. As with most of the movements for this gait you get used to timing this cue so that it becomes natural and eventually require much less concentration and effort. Again it is a tremendous benefit to learn to ride and cue on an experienced horse first.

One initial squeeze is often not enough, and you should continue rhythmically squeezing – and – releasing the canter cue in time with the planting of that outside hind hoof, until the horse is picking up a nice rolling canter. It will most likely not happen at once. Indeed it will most likely take many days, even weeks, of working this cue in the round pen for the horse to both understand exactly what you're asking for, and learn to lift himself into that gear with your additional weight on board. You will usually start feeling the occasional hitch as you work.

As with training any new activity I use the fundamentals of the four R's. As soon as I feel that very first hitch and roll of a canter stride I will stop the horse and reward his effort; give him a tiny break and then resume training. Right now just getting the horse to understand what you want and give you the lifting motion is an important start. It is your foot in the door and something concrete that you can build on. But many horses have a difficult time understanding the concept of

SPECIAL CONSIDERATIONS

There are reasons for the myth of not cantering your gaited horse as we discussed. The truth is that it ***can*** be very difficult for a gaited horse to find a quality canter because of poor posture and balance coupled with their natural multi-gaited abilities, added to the fact of being very forward horses. The common practice of framing up the gaited horse to find a smooth easy gait almost guarantees the likelihood that they will brace up their topline into a dorsal dominance, producing stiffness and encouraging heavy-on-the-fore carriage. The heaviness on the fore adds tremendous difficulty for lifting that fore when combined with a strung-out backend. Your horse needs this lift for an elegant and correct canter so this unbalanced carriage must be addressed first. See **Recommended Exercises above** for reconditioning and rebalancing your horse as a first step toward developing this very desirable gait.

Balance and conditioning are vital. Balance is every bit as important as strength to engage a quality canter with a rider on board and this is where many gaited horses have added difficulty. The dorsal dominant horse is starting out tremendously unbalanced. The shoulders support the entire front of his body and to get this off the ground he must engage his backend well beneath and utilize both dorsal and ventral muscling of his core. The stiffness and strung out backend associated with hollow carriage inhibits both the coiling and the lifting movements he needs. It is this incorrect posture that makes an effortless canter very difficult for these horses to accomplish, and most likely why gaited horses

us wanting them to canter, especially if we've been riding them for a long time without asking for this gear. You must be persistent and patient. He will get it....eventually.

as a whole have such an undeserved reputation for being difficult to train in canter. It takes all these muscles working in concert to gather under, plant and lift up the fore.

We must own up and place the blame for the difficulty many gaited horses experience in finding a correct canter right where it belongs; squarely on our own shoulders for not understanding how the poor equitation has set our horses up to fail in this, their final finished gait. We must first help the horse find a posture that is not only conducive to a quality canter but condition the needed muscles to allow the gait with much less strain.

While an initial strong push-off from the shoulder is essential, it must be coupled with the balance to coil the croup, allowing the engaged backend to power-lift the front into the lead. ***A lifting of the fore/base of the neck/shoulder is what allows the backend to coil beneath to plant and drive the gait.*** Without this essential lightness and lift the backend cannot properly engage and will tend to string out behind. When this happens the gait alters; becomes flatter, faster and out of balance with the horse feeling as though he's throwing himself forward rather than deliberately lifting and rolling back down. This lift cannot be artificially forced by pulling on the head through the mouth with the reins; and indeed that action will create the opposite hollow core posture we need to overcome. The horse must shift his balance by rounding his core as he pushes off with his shoulders using his head and neck in a lifting motion to assist his upward push. This lift then enables a necessary coiling of the loins to bring his hind legs under to drive this gait rather than simply pushing forward as the strung-out hindquarters do.

This balance and use of the body is why a canter is the best gait for horses to execute jumps and why many trainers recommend using a small walkover pole to help the horse find the attitude initially. While the head and neck will provide assistance with both the rebalance and the lift, *it must be initiated from the horse and never forced from the rider.* When the horse is hollow and out of balance, we see riders resort to severely pumping on the reins in attempt to pull the horse up into his canter. *Please understand* it can't be done so don't go there! Pumping the reins not only produces a very hollow, awkward and uncomfortable looking gait that is painful to watch, it also demonstrates that you're trying to force a movement that your horse is not in proper balance to perform.

It is of further note that as most horses first begin cantering under saddle they often exhibit a preference of one lead over another. This is completely typical, and should be expected. After all most of us have a stronger tendency to use one side of our body over another, with only a small percentage being completely and equally ambidextrous. Once the horse understands how to pick up the gait on his preferred side, I begin working on the opposite lead and *will work that weaker side at least twice as much as the stronger lead.* Our goal should always be to develop a balanced and straight horse, which includes being able to carry this non-symmetrical gait evenly on both sides. After asking and getting a few quality strides on the strong lead, I immediately turn the horse in the arena or round pen to work on the weaker lead. If the horse starts showing evidence of frustration or just doesn't seem to get it on the weaker lead, I work the rounding exercises and the slow, deep walking for a few minutes to give them a break before again asking for the weak lead. I will also reverse the horse and

pickup the strong lead again for a few strides so that I may stop and reward their effort and let them end on a good note. Remember this is a conditioning and strengthening **project,** and gaited horses that pick up the canter automatically and effortlessly when first asked are not as common as I would hope. So plan to spend a few weeks building strength and coordination of movement before you begin seeing that nice hitch and roll that can later be polished into the elegant canter we all love. If it happens quicker, then you should feel blessed and kiss your horse for being such a brilliant and willing partner.

When you have established the canter cue and your horse is beginning to respond to it with at least the effort of lifting into canter, you must remember to transition to riding the canter movement as described in step 4, until such time as the horse starts to fall out of the canter or you decide to leave that gait. If the horse starts to fall out of gait before you are ready, you need to once again pick up the driving cue in rhythm. Learn to go passive while he's moving correctly, moving with the gait, then transition back to the more aggressive driving seat should he start to fall out of gait.

The exception of course, is when the horse is first learning. Most will be very close to falling forward into the pace-gallop as they pick up those first careful strides. To help counter the tendency to fall forward you will need to *always be mindful of your speed and build this gait a few strides at a time while maintaining the slower, controlled tempo.* As the horse lifts and rolls into his first efforts of canter it will be most natural for him to want to continue increasing his speed. Proper form for this gait means *speed is the enemy* and will cause him to lose both form and balance every time. This is one of the primary reasons for starting it from a walk speed and keeping it at walking tempo. The very dynamic of a horse pushing *up* rather than forward is what helps him maintain proper form. Remember that lateral timing supports a more forward movement while the more diagonal timing supports lift and upward movements. We need our horse to keep his backend engaged and his core neutral to slightly round in support of a quality canter.

After the horse has learned to carry the slow rolling deep canter you can always ask him to extend it with just a bit of practice, but the slow roll is going to be his biggest challenge and *REQUIRE THE MOST STRENGTH, BALANCE AND CONTROL.* You need your horse to disassociate the canter cue from the gallop cue. HE needs to comprehend you're not asking for speed. Pay attention and as soon as you feel him tilt to throw himself forward he's losing form and you will need to use a half-halt to resist and correct. He needs to *KEEP THE MOTION SLOW, DELIBERATE, BALANCED AND LIFTING* to maintain.

Once you get your horse to lift into two strides of canter, stop him and reward. Repeat this process and again only ask for two strides of canter and stop to reward. Don't keep going until he falls out of form. We do not want him to deliberately try to fall out so he can stop. You need to reward his correct motion, and stopping is part of that reward. Also we want to reward correct movement not incorrect, so if he does manage to fall out, we must immediately ask him to pick it up again.

It takes strength to maintain balance at the slower rolling canter and speed will never be an acceptable substitute. That first week he's hitching and lifting into gait I work only two strides at a time then stop, pause for reward, walk out and ask again. To ask for more will set him up to fail and fall out. The next week I will ask for three strides as long as he can do it without falling out of balance or throwing himself into the pace-gallop. Remember patience and persistence. I add a stride each week for the first month or two until he can carry it the length of the arena, then I begin adding at a faster rate which becomes a subjective call based on the size, age and condition of your horse, as well as the weight of the rider. He must build the muscles to support this balanced gait; so don't push it or you'll lose it.

WHY TROTTING HORSES CANTER EASIER

Diagonally timed gaits support more upward movement and loft, while more laterally timed gaits support more forward movement.

Most people recognize that there is a strong element of diagonal movement to a correct canter where the off lead diagonal pairs land together. One could conclude that the roundness of a collected core would support an easier pairing of those non-lead diagonal pairs.

It also makes sense that the roundness already present through his core when carrying more diagonally timed gait allows the dorsal muscles to share the needed lift with the haunch muscles for the a cantering horse (see EXERCISE in the next section). Let me explain this correlation. Pacing horses whose dorsal muscles are *ALREADY CONTRACTED* due to their dorsal dominant carriage have very little additional pull with those muscles simply because there is nowhere further to go when they are already contracted. A muscle can only contract so far. Therefore, in an already dorsally dominant carriage the burden of all lifting must get shifted to the legs alone.

Also, as stated before, most pacers can out-pace the speed of a canter; therefore to attempt to train or encourage the canter as a progression of speed is illogical and rarely successful in a horse that readily finds a pace. While this is the method traditionally used for non-gaited breeds in training the canter, most gaited horses will simply pace harder. The only thing faster than a pace is an all-out gallop: flat, four beat and fast. Hmmm? Where have we heard that before? You even hear of stock horse trainers who advocate simply pushing a gaited horse into a gallop and keeping them there until they are exhausted and slow down into a canter or lope. This sounds like a hard way to train a horse and not too kind to the horse as well. Plus we have the significantly increased risk of hock and stifle strains if our gaited horse is very young. For these as well as numerous other reasons I will never advocate this method of finding a canter.

LAMENESS CONCERNS

I am absolutely convinced that there is a direct correlation between training a canter *WHEN HORSES (PARTICULARLY YOUNG HORSES) ARE MOVING HOLLOW* and a proliferation of stifle injuries and lumbosacral joint strains commonly seen in so many breeds. The frequency of these injuries has given gaited horses added reputation of being less sturdy, but I don't believe this is simply a case of poor conformation. I am convinced it is directly related to the practice of allowing, even encouraging, horses to travel hollow in dorsal dominance that is placing them in a fragile and unbalanced posture then asking for strong or fast hindquarter impulsion or lift. The very kind of impulsion needed for lifting into canter and for fast forward take off. This dorsal dominant posture disengages their core muscles from assisting the haunches in any strong maneuver such as picking up a canter. While I will not lay 100% of the blame for hindquarter lamenesses on the hollow core posture, I believe it contributes significantly.

We expose ourselves to a similar weakness as we lift a heavy load and strain our backs by bending only at the waist. As we learn to squat for the lift we share the load with our legs and significantly lessen the risk of back strain. By altering our posture in preparation we have reduced the strain because the burden is no longer isolated to only one group of muscles but shared among many.

Similarly, when a horse carries himself dorsal dominant with their croup already uncoiled they have taken the core support out of the picture as well. This posture significantly increases the strain on the muscles and joints of the hindquarters as well as the sacrum as a horse lifts his weight into the canter or accelerates abruptly. In dorsal dominant posture those muscles are disconnected from sharing the load or needed power because they are already contracted almost to maximum.

EXERCISE: *Stand with your feet shoulder width apart and lean back slightly so that your shoulders are aligned 2-3 inches behind your pelvis. Now give a small jump or hop while your back is arched in this manner. Feel how little upward push you can get when you take your core muscles out of play; how all the strain of the hop gets placed squarely on your leg and thigh muscles. Now come forward to align your shoulders slightly in front of your pelvis and try hopping again. Feel how your back muscles contract to assist this small lofting motion and you'll begin to understand how important it is to share the load as well as the push with your core muscles.*

I use this exercise to illustrate how a hollow/dorsal dominant posture ***disconnects*** the core and places all the strain onto the hind legs of a horse that's trying to lift himself into a canter.

This assertion of a connection between hollow carriage to stifle and lumbosacral strains comes mostly from my own observations. There are multiple studies that confirm dressage and jumping horses, while strung out behind, have a propensity toward hunter's bump resulting from LS joint strain. I feel this strain is caused by this same disconnect of core muscles. By helping horses learn to release their hollow posture, lift and round their core shifts and shares the burden of any athletic maneuver between more muscles. This along with conditioning and strengthening both the haunch and core muscles may help avoid a strain with its related lameness, scar tissue and future off-stride. When a horse learns to properly engage his core the lift into canter the maneuver becomes much easier. When he builds his haunch and core muscles slowly to accommodate carrying a rider in this gait it becomes quite effortless in a relatively short amount of time and often a preferred gait for him.

This is just one more reason I strongly advise allowing yourself and your horse several weeks *OR EVEN MONTHS TO* condition and build into a correct canter. Even if you're blessed with a young horse that picks it up easily, please be cautious in limiting the time you ride the canter during those early weeks and months. Just as starting horses too young can have lasting consequences, especially in those breeds where looseness and long stride are desired, pushing too soon or too long at the canter can strain young joints and increase the likelihood of injury. The joints of young horses are delicate until they quit going through growth spurts somewhere between 5 ½ and 7 years old. While most of these injuries will heal, it is common that the range of motion in those healed joints may be forever compromised and limited by scar tissue with less elasticity than the original and undamaged cartilage. This lack of elasticity results in shortened and off strides along with unbalanced gaits.

Injuries such as these will also increase the likelihood of arthritis later in the horse's life as well. Care should be taken to maintain good orthopedic posture and attitudes for increased longevity. This is particularly true when training the canter because it is an asymmetrical gait that places more strain on one side than the other.

While this is not only a gaited horse issue it is an issue for gaited horses. We not only see a preponderance of lumbosacral strains and hunters' bumps but a multitude of stifle and hock injuries as well. Close observation will often reveal a preponderance of shortened stride on one side or the other in a significant sampling of gaited horses. Before we can draw the conclusion of poor breeding, we must first own up to poor training practices.

LEAD CHANGES

When you remain clear with your cue and consistent in how you ask for a canter your horse becomes more and more comfortable with effortlessly and readily picking it up. Eventually he will almost seem to read your mind and may even try to anticipate your cues by your unconscious preparation. This clarity and consistency also sets you up for eventually moving on to the flying lead changes. But I will caution that learning to consistently cue in correct timing is probably the greatest challenge for riders new to this gait, and until you feel you are polished enough with both cues and riding both leads of the canter I would advise dropping down to the walk for a couple of strides, get your timing correct, then picking up the canter fresh in the new lead. Called a simple lead change, practicing this canter-walk-canter transition will help you become so familiar with the cue that you will avoid a lot of confusion and possibly frustration on the part of your horse as you advance to the flying changes. Please don't blame the horse if you are new to lead changes. Everybody is allowed their learning curve, even riders. Take your time and everyone will be happier for it.

I recommend when you are ready to go for the flying lead change you use an approach of cantering through a figure "8" and holding the initial lead until your horse has crossed the center and counter-cantering on the opposite curve. Only then ask for your lead change.

THE CROSS-FIRE CANTER

If you've never heard of this particular problem, then count yourself lucky. A cross-fire canter is where the back supporting pair of legs are on one lead and the fore legs are on the other lead. While a normal canter is called a transverse canter where the legs are used in alternating sides, the cross-fire canter is called a rotational canter indicating the way the legs are being used in a circular cycle. Watching from the ground a quick telltale of the crossfire is the lateral pairs will either be on opposite extremes or next to each other. The lead leg and the driving leg will be on the same side of the body with the legs on the other (lateral) side landing closely together, appearing between the outstretched and widely separated driving and lead legs.

If you have a horse that attempts to switch into crossfire while training it will often feel so rough as to almost unseat you. It is very abrupt and the action of switching can feel quite violent. However I have seen horses that appear to consistently crossfire seamlessly, and obviously they are more comfortable in the crossfire. Those horses should be checked for back and leg problems that are commonly found in horses that routinely carry the crossfire.

When I witness a cross-fire canter I immediately seek to determine if there is a physical problem. It is my experience that most cross-fire canters are a result of pain or discomfort that can often be traced to a current or past lameness or back injury. Your initial responsibility is to determine if the horse is

When counter-cantering your horse wants to quite naturally change leads to accommodate the curve of the figure "8". This sets him up for success. It allows your horse to learn to change leads on the fly, but you will still need to practice YOUR timing and cue.

sound enough to carry a correct, transverse driving canter. The next is to NOT allow him to carry this incorrect cross-fire canter. Resolve any physical issues first if at all possible then slowly and patiently train a correct canter take off from a walking speed.

Closely observe which hind leg is driving the cross-fire, or if it occurs on both leads. I have seen horses favor lamenesses by switching behind and driving off the wrong back leg to compensate for discomfort and protect a weaker limb. When this is observed it tells me to look to the non-driving hind as the likely source for the problem. If the cross-fire is limited to only one lead it increases the likelihood of a lameness located somewhere in the leg that should be driving that lead and which the horse is switching to avoid stressing.

I further recommend examining the flatfoot walk closely for evenness of stride, fluid use of the headnod which should *BE EQUALLY DEEP AS EACH HIND LEG PLANTS AND EQUALLY HIGH AS EACH FORELEG PLANTS*. Further examination for possible back pain would be advised for horses that are consistently unable to pick up and maintain the correctly transverse canter. Sometimes slowing down the canter cue to a slow walking tempo will help the horse avoid the crossfire if they are using it to protect a weaker limb from extreme acceleration. In either case please have a veterinarian conduct a complete lameness exam to check for possible issues.

Part IV – A NATURALLY BRILLIANT WALKING HORSE

Truly brilliant movement comes from within the horse. A knowledgeable rider can help his horse tap into his balance and impulsion; he can ask the horse for bigger, better, deeper, longer and overall more. But True Natural Brilliance only occurs when the horse reaches into himself and offers it to his rider. It can *NEVER* be forced, framed, fixed or nailed on.

Those who see performance as their ultimate goal must make a choice about what kind of trainer/rider/owner they want to be and work with their horse accordingly. If they admit that the blue ribbon is the most vital goal they are likely to be willing to employ some level of mechanical enhancements to get there. Or you may be one who chooses to strive for a superior partnership and level of communication that encourages your horse to give more of himself to please you, his riding partner. This chapter is for those who choose the latter of these alternatives.

I see so much that is wrong with the performance training of show horses that I simply could not publish any book without addressing the tremendous need within the gaited horse industry to evolve beyond the current fix it mentality that is so common and widely accepted. Because of the biggest is best attitude when it comes to training and yes, to judging as well, the Walking Horse as a breed has been cheated of the chance to improve through strictly athletic training, conditioning and breeding. The TWH community seems to have jumped off the progressive track to evolve somewhere around 1949-1950. We moved away from sound and ethical breeding, training and exhibition to go for the mechanical fix that is not really a fix at all.

Far too much of the current training and judging rewards whoever rides into the ring with the biggest front end and the biggest backend even if the gait no longer resembles what these horses were founded and celebrated for. Current judging practices seem based on erroneous ideas of overstride and how close a back hoof plants to the opposite front; both measurements which I have shown to be firmly in the *MYTH CATEGORY*.

Trainer Gary Lane and I discuss on our DVD TRAINING THE GAITED HORSE, while using split screen comparisons, how naturally trained Walking Horses today still have the abilities and the genetics to produce those foundation gaits. So why are these gaits no longer being rewarded by a majority of the judges at shows? Maybe because they've been deemed not flashy enough; not fast and not big enough. Well sorry to burst some bubbles, but the flash and speed were not the goals that produced these horses in the first place. It is their energy efficient, smooth riding, relaxed gait plus their sensible mind and willing heart, making them the number one pleasure horse option out there today. All the foundation characteristics are what riders of today want for their trail pleasure partners, not the flash and speed. That is why the popularity of the Saddlebreds appears to be in decline while the popularity of the Walking Horse is escalating. People want a horse they can shine up and show on Saturday night, then relax as they hit the trail with on Sunday afternoon.

But this is not to say that we cannot have an exciting show horse built from the inherent talent within. In my years of training I have shown that proper posture and balance coupled with wet saddle pad time can and does produce a natural brilliance that is both eye catching and beautiful for those who have the sense to see it. We are fortunate that there are now show circuits and venues available for those of us who want to celebrate these natural abilities and brilliance; both circuits and judging programs that embrace and reward these amazingly talented animals for their athletic accomplishments, not their ability to carry appliances. The walking gaits as well as the rocking chair canter are a thing of beauty when offered and developed to a higher level by a horse who's shod sensibly or even barefoot, and has developed a strong backend to float a brilliant front end. It has nothing to do with weight, angle, hoof bands, action devices or stacks. Those are tools for the uninformed and unwilling to evolve.

A personal note here is that while I have developed horses to a high level of performance, and done so naturally, I do not believe in competing at any events that hire HIO's that do not ACTIVELY SUPPORT the USDA's efforts to clean up the show industry of the Tennessee Walking Horse and the Spotted Saddle Horse. It's an embarrassment for those of us who love these horses to have this blight on their reputation and as testament to the lack of true horsemanship that has been commonly accepted by those in charge of those HIO's.

We, as exhibitors choose who we support and who we show with and who makes money from our horses. I may have to drive a little further, spend an extra night away from home to show with those HIO's who actively protect the horse, but those are the only ribbons worth winning. ***Quite frankly, how we spend our money is the only real voice we have in this industry, so please use your voice wisely***.

I will also say that you should never define yourself or your horse by the show ring. To do so does him and you a disservice. Showing your horse should be a hobby only. It should be just another way to enjoy and celebrate the partnership you have with him and to socialize with others who feel the same. Don't ever give a show or a judge the power to make you feel less than delighted with the relationship you've built with your equine partner. He/she can only judge the ring on that day, that moment and for those specific attributes and you should never take their momentary opinion as an indictment of your horse.

Chapter 13 - Performance Formula

I imagine many people may well turn to this chapter thinking they're going to read a recommendation for shoeing, bitting and riding in the show ring...not exactly. Within the following chapters is my formula for developing a ***naturally brilliant and showy walking horse*** that will find rewards in many show rings today; a formula that I personally feel is the future of the Tennessee Walking Horse. This is a formula developed from the horse's abilities and not what can be done *to* him.

I will tell you right now that there are (unfortunately) judges that will never appreciate the kind of natural brilliance that so many of us find compelling; they do not and will not appreciate those gaits that make my heart rise up with hope for the future of this breed in the show ring. There are show circuit judges that will gauge only two things when horses enter the ring: overstride of the backend and break of the front hooves (the fold and lift of the knee and fetlock). They glance to see the overstride and gauge how closely each hind foot plants to its opposite fore, without any consideration for the critical timing component of those measurements. In the following chapters I will show how both of these are man-made and faulty criteria for judging correct walking gait and *SHOULD NOT BE A CONSIDERATION OF ANY JUDGE WHO KNOWS WHAT HE OR SHE SHOULD BE LOOKING TO REWARD.*

My experience is that if you can get your horse correct and consistent in his gait you are halfway toward a blue ribbon in those show circuits and HIOs that promote *CORRECT GAIT OVER ANIMATION*. Before it can be big and showy it must be correct!

I find that TRUE brilliance in the show ring comes from 3 things: Strong Impulsion from a driving backend; looseness; and freedom of the head for gait 'expression'. While the first two will be limited somewhat by your horse's conformation, the third is completely in your hands (forgive that pun).

A strong driving backend being carried with a neutral topline allowing the energy to flow through will express itself as a bloom in the front. This bloom is a fluid lightness and float of the front end that maintains the roll and reach of the shoulders while allowing the headnod to productively power the driving backend. It's a beautiful picture when correctly produced from lightness and engagement. It has NOTHING to do with what shoes are on the front hooves, or how much the knees and fetlocks fold and lift. *MECHANICAL AIDS HONESTLY DEGRADE A TRUE AND CORRECT GAIT RATHER THAN ENHANCE IT.* When a trainer, owner or rider chooses to go down the path of mechanical enhancements the gait changes significantly and becomes much more stiff and laborious for the horse. A mechanically enhanced horse appears jerky, tight and has lost his forward flow. When extreme weight is added in attempt to force animated motion of the front hooves the backend must compensate, usually with an artificial squat that causes the hocks to rotate in a very unnatural manner that I find obscene and extremely difficult to watch. But we will continue to see people resort to these machinations as long as we have judges with authority and inclination to reward them.

Of further note is that in order to usher our beloved breed into the new arena of NATURAL BRILLIANCE, we must learn and be able to identify and differentiate that which is manmade from that which is natural to and from the horse. While those within the traditional industry must learn to train and develop a different type of horse, those within the sound horse community must not let our aversion of all things mechanical cause us to shy away from asking our horses to get bigger and do more. As long as we are asking the horse to offer unenhanced physical effort why not give him the months and years (yes years) to develop his athletic abilities? We know and expect a human athlete to work to condition himself for many years, so it makes no sense to expect our horses to just spontaneously have this brilliance within a few weeks of training.

If we cannot open the door to this new arena for naturally talented competition for all to see and participate in WE WILL HAVE A MUCH HARDER TIME CLOSING OFF THE OLD ARENA OF MECHANICAL INFLUENCES AND ENHANCEMENTS. We need to embrace and welcome those who love these horses to work with them to breed for and achieve a much higher level of gait just as a warm blood can be brought to a higher level of dressage maneuvers, through the honest sweat of both horse and rider.

BALANCE AND ENGAGEMENT

Your primary goal should always be to first get your horse correct, then build his gaits from that correct carriage. His walking gait, posture and timing should be established at the trail walk speed as even, loose and working all four corners equally balanced. His head should nod along with his stride in relaxation with a soft front-to-back roll beneath the saddle that pushes your hips along with it. This is your horse's initial DEFAULT GAIT which is the gear you will always want to come back to when you feel things going wrong.

You, as trainer of your horse, need to learn to *feel his movement through your seat*. It is tremendously helpful to learn the feel of his sweeping backend stride and understand when it's engaged and driving properly or when it's bracing, shortening and disengaging.

Your own hips should sweep front-to-back SYMMETRICALLY as evidence that your horse is even and straight in his stride. If you have doubts about what you feel, take time for some relaxed riding in an enclosed area such as an arena or round pen. Ride slowly while closing your eyes to better focus on the FEEL. Learn the correct movements so that you'll be able to identify when he is correct and when he begins to change. Learn the feel of each leg movement of your horse's stride *through your own core*. When riding with a balanced and independent seat you should have a released lumbar area that allows your hips and legs to move with your horse while keeping your shoulders and head level and quiet.

Hint: your hips should move in alternating but equal front-to-back rolling movements, while your chest, shoulders and head remain level and quiet. <u>*If you feel a lifting through your own shoulders then most likely your horse has disengaged his hindquarters and is beginning to loft through his backend by tightening his hips and engaging his hocks.*</u> *You need to feel when this occurs and correct him to re-establish hindquarter engagement.*

There should never be any lifting or lofting only sweeping movement from the backend while executing correct walking gaits. At the moment you feel loft your horse has begun to suspend during the backend weight transfer. Some mistakenly consider this appropriate because they are so used to riding the racking gaits on their pleasure horses. There is nothing wrong with a rack if that is what you want and what you like. If, however, you wish to develop a Walking Horse for show you will need to keep him driving and sweeping with this backend. Loft is not allowed, or at least will be penalized by any knowledgeable judge simply because it tells us the horse is no longer using his hindquarters correctly. From the ground the tail dock can be seen to have a soft side-to-side swing or waggle as he sweeps his strides. That same tail dock will begin jigging with suspension if or when he disengages his striding sweep into a suspended and jogging step.

HEADNOD

HEAD MOVEMENT IS AN 'EXPRESSION' OF WHATEVER GAIT IS BEING CARRIED BY A HORSE.

The headnod of a walking gait is the surest indication that your horse is remaining in form and using himself correctly. If the headnod disappears or changes dramatically your horse has most likely braced at the shoulders or has engaged his dorsal muscles with tension in likely preparation for increased speed. Either of these indicates degradation or a complete change of gait away from a true walk. As we described in the early chapters on biomechanics a walk is defined by the fluidity of a topline carried in neutral posture with rolling hips and shoulders. All this fluid looseness allows for non-suspended weight transfer both front and back. If any of these characteristics change so does the gait. Existing together you will invariably see an up and down nodding of the head as the driving energy of the backend flows through the horse unimpeded to the poll for expression. It is vital that the headnod originate at the shoulder or base of the neck. You should easily be able to identify that the angle of alignment from neck to back is alternating with the stride. Two up and down nods occur for each complete rotation and are in synchronization with his back hooves.

When you see the headnod starting to diminish you should first ask the horse to return to his loose, neutral carriage by lower his head and give at his poll for a more vertical head carriage, then *IMMEDIATELY RELEASE HIM WHEN HE GIVES.* Both these movements encourage him to telescope his neck and back vertebrae, and to release back into neutral posture.

As his rider and trainer it is important that you allow him the freedom to use his head and stay out of his way. Keep your hands low, positioned quietly on either side of his withers with your elbows fixed at your side and your forearms angled toward the bit.

Please note that both disengagement of the backend as well as losing the headnod are strong indicators that the horse is balancing more heavily toward his fore. This is an all too common problem, and is more likely to occur the faster a horse is asked to move. As a horse increases the tension in his shoulders, head and neck the headnod begins to subside. Not only does the tension promotes a tendency to sink somewhat at the base of his neck and lose his lightness of the front but it also blocks the fluid flow of energy from the backend stride that powers the headnod. This tension through the shoulders head and neck, along with backend disengagement are natural occurrences of heavy on the fore balance, and both can usually be solved by a rebalancing of the horse toward the hindquarters. Both are symptoms of front-to-back imbalance rather than individual issues to be corrected. *THIS FURTHER ILLUSTRATES WHY BALANCE IS CRITICAL*

FOR A QUALITY FLATFOOT WALK, AND MUST BE MAINTAINED FOR YOUR HORSE TO INCREASE HIS

Rating your horse

Once you learn to ride with your horse's movement in a passive seat you can begin learning to influence his movement with an active seat. I love this wonderful quote from Ray Hunt's book <u>THINK HARMONY WITH HORSES</u> and just couldn't resist inserting here also. It's appropriate in so many ways.

"A walk is a four beat gait and should be regular. You should be able to control it. If you want him to walk a little faster, you reach a little further with your legs, with your fanny, with the soles of your feet and the seat of your britches, with your MIND, with your positive thinking. You are picking his feet up and setting them down. You're going with him so he can learn to go with you – feel it. See how little it takes to do the job. If you can put you reins on the horn, fold your arms and he will do it --- that's what you will do. Its feel, timing and balance. It can become as natural as breathing."

I think this quote perfectly captures the need for feeling your horse and teaching him to feel and rate to you. It's not difficult to tell people to become one with their horse and to move in harmony, but it does take patient effort to learn the skill of feeling, following then directing with your seat and legs. It is particularly helpful to communicate on this level with any horse that is high strung or nervous because any excess rein contact tends to increase their anxiety and agitation. If you can learn to communicate more with your seat and legs, using lighter and less rein contact, it often allows many of these high strung horses to relax and calm to a huge degree at which point they can both think better and listen closer.

Before you can ask your horse to extend his reach, you must be able to influence and

SPEED TO EXTEND INTO A CORRECT RUNNING WALK.

direct his tempo. This ability to establish, maintain and synchronize his tempo (to rate) to your seat is extremely critical step toward developing a big, bold and brilliant show gait.

For many high-strung horses you'll need to emotionally connect with them by first moving with their rolling front to back movement with a more passive seat. I recommend using only subtle nudges of your calves while tilting and rolling through your pelvis. I've heard some ladies say this feels weird and slightly obscene going with that pelvic roll, but I say "get over it!" Your job is to ride and communicate with your horse so he can understand what you want while maintaining an independent seat and not interfering with his natural movement. If you want to be prim and proper in the way you ride, maybe you should consider getting a racking horse to sit in a quiet chair seat. If, conversely, you want to get the best walk out of your horse you will need *TO MOVE WITH HIM AND ENCOURAGE HIS WALKING MOTION.* What many don't realize is that if you don't move with your horse you are actually communicating resistance to him. Unlocking your lumbar area and moving with the natural and correct movement of your horse is just one more way of encouraging and telling him he is doing what you want.

I love to play up-beat music in my barn while I'm riding. I have put together a CD with a variety of pieces that I like with different tempos and as the music changes I challenge my horse to rate his tempo to the new rhythm. This gives me a focus for this exercise and a way of knowing that he is going with me rather than me going with him. There can only be one leader of any dancing couple and many horses really want that leading roll. I have flatfoot walk music, running walk (and fox trotting) music, canter music and racking music. It's great to challenge both yourself and your horse while learning to communicate with him on this level, all the while trying not to manipulate him through the reins-and-hands-to-mouth. This exercise will make you a better rider at the same time that it trains your horse to listen closer to you.

THE GOAL: Once you have your horse listening and rating himself to your seat it's time for the next level. You want to *GET BIGGER WITHOUT GETTING FASTER.* You want to subtly encourage your horse to increase his energy, his reach and his stride while keeping his tempo slow and even. This is how you'll teach him to *LENGTHEN HIS STRIDE NATURALLY*, without resorting to mechanical influences. PLEASE RE-READ RAY'S QUOTE ABOVE! This is as much a mental exercise for you as it is with your horse. You need to THINK him bigger, FEEL him bigger and RELEASE him into bigger stride.

Don't be at all surprised if at first your horse wants to speed up rather than extend … actually you should expect it. Just patiently check his tempo and try again. Rating his speed is one new concept while learning to extend his stride and energy without accelerating his rhythm is another. Remember it's important to reward your horse if you feel a particularly light and brilliant few strides that indicates he's making a good faith effort to adjust his carriage. Sometimes that's all you'll get at first. When you feel lightness, stop him, stroke him and tell him what a good boy he is, then try again. I even like to keep some small nibble treats in my pockets for just such moments because it's a great way to get across to your horse that he just grasped a particularly challenging concept. Be careful to not overuse the treat reward… you don't want him deliberately stopping for a food every few steps. Your challenge is to help your horse to find his deepest and boldest walk while maintaining a consistently slower, marching tempo. You'll always be able to

extend his speed once you have the deep walk, but that is down the road.

We're helping your horse build his running walk from the brilliant and solidly four-cornered flatfoot walk. The better his flatfoot walk the better his running walk can and will be. I frequently see horses that will exhibit a brilliant slower walk, but will dramatically lose form as they speed up. The nature of increasing speed encourages more tension which ultimately changes their balance and fluidity. It's common to see horses actually shorten their stride and border on disengaging the backend as they transition to the running walk because they have not been trained in the deep flatfoot walk long enough to establish it as the foundation walking gait, or because the rider is asking them to accelerate too quickly for them to maintain balance and form. If you want to show your horse *THE BEST THING YOU CAN DO IS INVEST THE NECESSARY TIME TO ESTABLISH THIS DEEP AND EVEN FLATFOOT WALK* to build on as you bring up his speed. Establish it firmly into his muscle memory by repetition and conditioning.

Once you have this deep reaching flatfoot walk well established with your horse and he is following your lead for tempo and speed, begin encouraging a slow transition up to the running walk. I say slow because if you cue the transition too fast your horse will most likely try to change gears rather than extend the gear he's in. We want to encourage him to *REV HIS ENGINE RATHER THAN CHANGE HIS GEAR,* and this requires subtle encouragement for extending the flatfoot walking gait. Just one more reason for training yourself and your horse to rate his tempo to your seat and legs is that it gives you the tools to extend into the running walk. Remember not to ask for top speed right away. Extend a little and bring him back down. Do this again and again, then in a few days extend it a little more and bring him down again. You need to feel his form remaining constant and always maintain the ability to bring his tempo back to the flatfoot walk. It's not at all unusual for a young horse to exhibit at shows in a slow deliberate flatfoot walk and a faster flatfoot walk, rather than the running walk. Remember every judge and show circuit asserts that *"form should NEVER be sacrificed for speed"*. Meaning that while they want to see two distinct speeds of walk exhibited, they'd much rather you maintain form than get into a race and start racking, pacing or trotting. The running walk will get bigger, faster and better with each year you ride it as long as you do not allow the horse to break form.

Chapter 14 - When the walks go wrong

NOTE: IF YOU HAVE NOT YET READ CHAPTERS ON "GIVE", "BIT TRAINING" AND "POWER STEERING" PLEASE DO SO BEFORE PROCEEDING.

I felt it was important to use this chapter to address some common misconceptions and frequent problems encountered with the walking gaits and in training for those gaits. Many of these have evolved from the training myths originating back to the fix-it methods of mechanical manipulation rather than from authentic training of the horse. Our gaited training has a lot to answer for in trying to sidestep solid equestrian principles in favor of the quick fix, and our horses have paid the price. It's time for that to stop.

COLLECTION VS. HEADSET

I want to impress upon you the tremendous difference between collection and headset, though many in the traditional Walking Horse world seem to be unaware of it.

Walking Horse owners have long been told to "*set his head and collect 'im up!*" and far too many of us were willing to try it for a while. After all, isn't that what the Walking Horse bit was designed to do? But what is collection, and how much of it does my Walking Horse really need? What does headset do for him and why?

Pardon me for giving you my take on this sage bit of wisdom but I believe headset for the Walking Horse has become popular as a shortcut tool to break up a lateral two-beat pace into a not-quite-so-lateral four beat stepping pace, in both pleasure and performance horses. The perpetrators of this very mechanical manipulation use it to encourage a racky lift and fold in the front feet, increasing the arc of those feet, slowing their placement and allowing the back feet to plant first. This breaks up the pace timing of the lift creating a smooth but racky, stepping pace placement; adding to that is the snappy fold and lift that is flashier for the show ring. Wow, a two-fer! But this is NOT real collection! I've often wondered if they just don't know any better, or are attempting to somehow legitimize their riding technique by calling it that, but nothing could actually be further from the truth.

I consider collection on a scale from light to high collection depending on how many of the three spinal arches are involved and to what extent. True collection is _not_ a product of pulling in the headset, or framing up a horse. It actually has nothing to do with forced face position. It's something that is *given* by the horse when asked for, and should never be forced or held in by the rider. Collection comes from *self-carriage*; a gathering of the horse's body starting at the hocks, all the way through to the poll. The horse must *pull himself in* to offer the rider balanced impulsion for forward, upward or lateral movement

You should try to learn the feel of collection from the backend forward. First the loins must coil under as the sacrum is pulled inward and engaged down. Next the core (thoracolumbar arch) is released and rounded from the contraction of the abdominal (ventral) muscles, and finally the neck (cervical arch) should be gracefully arched from the WITHERS ALL THE WAY THROUGH THE POLL IN A CONTINUOUS LINE indicating the lower neck is lifted upward by the hammock style muscles under the neck and aided by his flex at the poll.

I illustrate true collection by using the analogy of a little league baseball player. His first time up to bat, his coach must help him position his body to attempt a proper swing at the ball. He will most likely stand flat footed, with straight legs and core while he tries to swing the bat in a level motion. Now flash forward a couple of years to this same little leaguer. He has learned to flex at the knees, balance forward on the balls of his feet, shifting his weight back away from the approaching ball and leaning his upper torso forward in anticipation. He gathers himself to add power, smoothness, quickness and grace to his forward swing. This is similar to what your horse should do when collecting himself, as he prepares to engage in athletic endeavor.

The little league coach can position the batter's body all day, and still get a lifeless swing without much power. Something similar to this happens when a horse travels while being held into headset, and braced into a hollow spine carriage. He is actually being inhibited from finding real collection by the brute force being applied to his mouth. His hind legs get strung out and he not only has difficulty in maintaining a four-beat gait, but sacrifices balance and impulsion as well. Usually the rider *believes* he is collecting the horse by pulling his nose into vertical headset but this

is a complete myth. They've most likely been told that's how it's done, but unfortunately they are just rudely cramming the horse into the bit. Most riders that are pulling the head up in this manner can actually *cause* the spine to hollow out, which in turn *encourages* that pacing off-gait from their horse. It becomes a vicious catch-22 with the rider cramming the horse more and more until finally the horse begins moving his front feet in a rack and breaks into a stepping pace.

The physical effects of riding in this posture becomes a total picture for those that recognize the story it tells: weak, flat neckline in front of the withers; over-flexed muscles on either side of the poll with bulging resistance muscles down the front of the neck with the head held overly high for the horse's conformation. This is the infamous ewe or elk neck that in reality indicates that a horse is locked from jaw throughout their shoulders because his head is forced higher than his cervical vertebrae would naturally dictate. These horses are trying vainly to find relief from the overly severe bit leverage by trying to hold their mouth behind the bit. What we really should want and look for is a horse whose neck shows a nicely engaged arch from the withers forward to the poll indicating good self-carriage and allowing a natural rolling of their shoulders.

There is also the question of how much real collection we want and need in our Walking Horse? *Horses can and do move around all the time in a four-beat walk with absolutely no collection.* So the first thing you need to understand is that collection isn't *necessary* for a flatfoot walk or even the running walk for many horses. These are both neutral core carriage, balanced on all four corners gaits as most walks should be. Actually high collection involving all three spinal arches will probably push your Walking Horse into a nice jog trot. High collection occurs with significant rounding up through the core, with the pulling in of the loins through engagement of the croup as well as a lifting of the lower neck with the cervical arch. This is what the dressage horses are drilled for, but most of us don't want our Walking Horses moving in a trot. Upper level dressage involves maneuvers requiring upward loft and lightness.

Walking Horses preparing for the show ring only require light or minimal collection and then only when they have learned to carry a good flatfoot walk with no collection first. Light collection can add balance, grace and animation to the horse's carriage producing a more elegant stride while it promotes balanced impulsion. It further allows the front to get lighter and the energy produced by the backend to bloom into brilliance on the front. Again, it must be given by the horse and not framed by the rider through the bit. The horse needs to learn to carry the walking gait first to develop his muscle memory and to set his isochronal timing. He can then be asked to add light collection while maintaining that correct gait. He should keep neutral carriage through his core, neither hollowed nor rounded so neither core muscle groups dominate. This will help preserve the correct timing. You should encourage your horse to coil at the croup for backend engagement, as well as lifting the cervical arch for lightness at the withers as he gains speed. These balancing postures will support increased forward energy without losing form. This neck carriage will engage those muscles directly in front of the withers for proper lift and development allowing the headnod to work with more brilliance from the lifted lower neck. This is as much true collection as I recommend for any Walking Horse. To go beyond would be to interfere with their correct isochronal timing.

Care must be taken as you begin asking your horse to collect himself. Many Walking Horses will naturally be able to preserve the neutral core and maintain the even isochronal timing, but a few may tend to release and round that core and begin moving into a little more diagonally timed walk, possibly even flirting with a foxtrot that will push them toward disengagement of the croup as they morph nearer that alternate gait. When any gaited horse carries either dorsal or ventral dominance through his core the essential tension of those postures connects his front feet with his back feet and will push his gait more toward either a trot or a pace. Walking Horses working and showing in western disciplines with lower head on a loose rein *SHOULD NOT REQUIRE ANY COLLECTION AT ALL* other than a brief half-halt in preparation to execute more complex athletic maneuvers. To ask them for collection may well push them into a foxtrot while carrying their head and neck in the lower western positioning. Again, it's the horse doing the collecting, not the rider.

What I want to stress is that forcing false collection through a headset is the absolute last thing to do to actually *cure* the pace in a horse. Jamming the bit for headset creates many more problems than it solves, never mind the fact that the horse is off-gaited, stiff and uncomfortable to boot. I once had a mare brought to me for gait correction many years back that carried herself in just such a manor. Upon watching the owner ride her I quickly realized that *he* needed to learn as much as the mare. His hands were held high with an ten inch curb bit pulling the mare's head up even with *his* chest, while she traveled with a very short-strided and choppy pace, clearly more miserable than the rider. The first thing I did was put a snaffle bit on this mare and ask her to lower her head so the poll became level with her withers and round her neckline. Knowing from this posture she could more easily learn to find and keep her spine neutral. I could feel the tension immediately drain from her frame and hear her stride go to even timing as well as see the headnod start to develop. Within a couple of sessions she had softened her entire neckline and began to engage the bit, and with that engagement her stride went from a choppy pace to a nicely loose and correct flatfoot walk with 24 inches of overstride. On top of that I could feel her entire frame relax and noted that her eyes softened with comfort. While it takes horses like this many months to develop the muscles needed for this gait to become automatic and consistent, and it's up to the rider to resist any desire to pull the head high and push for speed, this posture will give a hollow horse the first opportunity to develop proper backend and strengthen the ventral muscles to carry the isochronal timing faster. Eventually these horses can be set well enough in this default gait to lift and carry their head wherever they wish without losing form. This

Overstride Illusion

Another leftover to be placed in the myth category is regarding the belief that overstride is a consistent method for evaluating the quality of a walking horse. We've all heard remarks about what *huge* overstride this or that horse has when observing their gait. Each time I hear remarks such as this I itch to open a debate about exactly what they believe overstride indicates. What I say here will surprise many because it is not commonly acknowledged, if even realized, in the traditional walking horse world though it should be.

Most within that industry will tell you that overstride (the point where a back hoof over-reaches the hoof print of the front hoof on the same side) is an accurate measurement of how long-strided a horse is. They also believe it is an accurate reflection of total stride length. What is not admitted or isn't realized is that *OVERSTRIDE IS ONLY AN ACCURATE MEASUREMENT FOR STRIDE COMPARISON WHEN ALL THE HORSES BEING COMPARED HAVE EXACTLY THE SAME PLACEMENT TIMING* to their gait. This, we all know, is quite rare indeed within walking horse show rings so why would they insist on using it? It is an illusion that they have bought

is one example of hundreds as I see this as the most common issue with gaited horses in general.

True, light collection can be a good thing in a Walking Horse when it's *OFFERED BY THE HORSE.* I hope I've illustrated that the false collection commonly seen with the elk neck is a flag for incorrect gait and uncomfortable as well as unbalanced posture, and that we should look for correct carriage and muscle definition in our Walking Horses. The old *"collect 'im up"* attitude using the infamous Walking Horse bit has done quite a disservice to the breed and riders as a whole. We need to move this bit of sage old wisdom into the myth category.

into.

Let me explain this inconsistency in detail. Using overstride to gauge and compare total stride will always be inaccurate and unreliable because of the influence of gait timing. Actual stride length is measured from the point where a hoof lifts off to where that same hoof plants again. When utilizing any factor that involves more than one hoof, timing becomes and essential part of the equation.

Furthermore, when a horse is moving more lateral (pacing or step-pacing) in his timing, he will consistently show a greater overstride than an evenly timed horse *WITH EXACTLY THE SAME AMOUNT OF STRIDE.* For that matter, the same horse with the same stride will show greater overstride when his gait moves to the lateral side of the spectrum and overstride will shorten as his gait moves to the diagonal side. Pacers will consistently show more overstride than more evenly timed or diagonally timed horses with *EXACTLY* the same total stride length. All overstride can really tell us is that a horse has decent stride and is reaching well in a sweeping walk.

If longer stride is truly the goal for breeding

quality walking horses then overstride should never be used as the defining gauge between horses with different timing. It is totally misleading, and is often used to fool gullible people into believing a horse has more reach than he really does. I personally believe that many trainers are fully aware that forcing a horse into a more lateral timing promotes this illusion and knowingly use it to fool others into believing that the horse has more stride than he actually does.

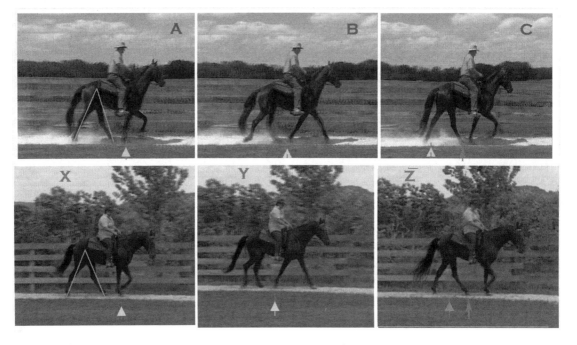

Figure 14.1 Peacemaker

Please study the series of photos above. This is *THE SAME HORSE IN THE SAME TACK ON THE SAME DAY, RIDDEN FIRST BY GARY LANE (ABOVE) AND BY MYSELF (BELOW) IMMEDIATELY AFTER.* Gary is *deliberately allowing* this horse to go to his default pace in photos A,B & C. While I am asking Peacemaker to drop his head, and release his dorsal dominant core. There are a number of things I wish to point out in comparison.

Gary Lane is a wonderful natural trainer who understands how important it is to achieve a lower head and natural even timing through the released topline for the pleasure horse. It is important to note that in these photos he is deliberately allowing this horse to go off-gait to better illustrate the differences in carriage and balance. Gary is showing us how Peacemaker currently defaults to a pace because at this point he had not advanced in his training to find a correctly neutral posture. Please visit WindSweptStables.net to find out more about Gary Lane and his natural training for the gaited horse.

Notice how high Peacemaker's head is in the upper shots where he is pacing. How his topline appears to be sunken at the shoulder demonstrating that he is balancing heavy on his fore as he paces. Conversely when he lowers his head and releases the topline he is more balanced front to back and not as sunken and heavy on the fore. The lower head carriage allows him to balance better. Though he has not yet achieved what I would classify as light on his front, he definitely *LESS HEAVY.*

Next I want to point out the angle of the backend stride in each of the starting photos,

A and X. If you compare just the backend reach in these two photos you'll see evidence that he is striding just as big in the walking sequence as he is in the pacing sequence. *SOME COULD ARGUE THAT HE IS ACTUALLY SHOWING A LITTLE DEEPER STRIDE AT THE WALK.* Again focus only on the backend and try not to involve the front in your measurement at this point.

Now finally look at the vertical lines I've marked below the front weight bearing hoof at each starting sequence. I've placed the same line to mark that place in each subsequent photo on both series, then as the sequence progresses you can see how far each back hoof over strides that mark as indicated with the second line I've added where his hind hoof plants and overstrides. The distance between these marks should illustrate how the pace timing at the top (lateral) produces a significantly greater overstride *measurement* than the more even (isochronal) timing on bottom produces. *A LONGER OVERSTRIDE IS BEING PRODUCED EVEN THOUGH WE'VE JUST POINTED OUT THAT HIS ACTUAL STRIDE IS EQUAL OR POSSIBLY EVEN GREATER AT THE WALK.* This is proof that overstride *cannot be used with any dependability as representative of actual stride length*, or even for comparison when judging horses at a show.

This thinking needs to be more commonly understood and accepted because I, or really anyone, can take a horse that would normally show an 18 inch overstride at his isochronal walk and push that horse into a pace or step-pace timing to produce a 26-30 inch overstride every time. The stride doesn't change and the horse is the same. The only thing that has changed is the timing which places that front hoof print further back in relationship to the overreaching back hoof. Simple geometry when you study it, really. Conversely I can take a pacing horse and square him, getting the same stride length at the walking gait and change that overstride back down to a more **accurate** 18 inches.

Timing and stride are not the only considerations of this measure, either. You must consider the additional factor that as a horse approaches a true two beat pace timing he may very well begin to loft between the lateral pairs of legs with a suspended weight transfer. That loft acts much like our jog and adds distance between the pickup and placement of a hoof. It transforms the nature of the stride being measured at that point from a true, non-suspended walk but becomes reach plus loft that includes a moment of aerial phase which further distorts the measurement.

The same flaw exists for those who would try to judge stride by comparing how closely a back hoof sets down to the opposite fore. Any time you are trying to make a comparison between more than one hoof, timing is an intricate part of the equation which should disqualify it as a reliable tool to measure or compare horses. An extremely well trained eye may take both overstride and timing into consideration but it takes careful study and becomes much more difficult at speed.

If it's all about stride then we need to bring our focus back to how much *actual* reach a horse has, and the only sure method is *MEASURING FROM THE POINT WHERE A HOOF LIFTS OFF TO THE POINT WHERE THAT SAME HOOF PLACES AGAIN AT A WALKING, NON-SUSPENDED STEP.* If stride is an important consideration for you, don't be fooled by miss-timed overstride into thinking that a horse is reaching bigger than he really is.

Actual stride measurements will vary greatly within this breed. But a brilliant extended stride in a Walking Horse will reach from 8 – 10 feet from pick up to set down. Many judges have accurately trained their eyes to gauge the angle produced by either supporting pair of legs but particularly the angle of the back leg stride. If you can train your eye to see this angle, in my mind it is a much better gauge of reach for any horse than his actual stride. For instance how can we reward a 17 hand horse for striding bigger than a 15 hand horse? His stride *should* be bigger because he has longer legs. However, many times the reach of the smaller horse will be greater *RELATIVE TO HIS SIZE* and to me should be more desirable if that is the characteristic being judged. The only way to gauge this accurately for comparison is to judge the angle produced between the legs of a supporting pair during the moment of weight transfer.

The huge stride of a walking horse is what takes the flatfoot walk and the running walk and produces a unique and brilliant gait that is both smooth to ride while efficiently covering the ground. Other breeds can be trained to a running walk, but only the Walking Horse, with their big stride and loose movement make a show of it.

Chapter 15 - Showing the Pleasure Walking Horse

I wish to talk about the vast differences that are produced and seen in horses trained naturally versus horses that have been trained using mechanical manipulations. The foundation Walking Horses were bred to be utility horses, but as they moved into the show arenas the unscrupulous owners, and desperate trainers started seeking quick methods for producing bigger and faster gaits to keep the attention of fans who were used to watching the flashy strides of the Saddlebreds at those very same shows. Once upon a time horses like Strolling Jim and Haynes Peacock were prized for their bold yet energy efficient and smooth riding gaits. Later, however, horses like Midnight Sun and Talk of the Town set the show world on fire with their brilliantly showy form that started upping the ante in that environment.

Rather than advancing abilities through hard work and saddle time as the horses in the dressage world commonly do, the walking horse industry began looking for shortcuts that would save time as well as years of saddle work to produce a showy gait. The problems inherent with this path are far too many to list, but even more than much of it being abusive and forceful with a horse, it means throwing away any opportunity that horse has to work in willing partnership. Also the mechanical manipulations embraced in the now traditional show training mask conformation deficiencies and create an environment where

breeders seek to produce horses that adapt to those mechanics rather than actually improve the breed through natural selection of solid conformational abilities. As a result the walking horses have only progressed in breeding qualities on a strictly hit and miss basis.

Bottom line, if anyone suggests using anything mechanical to *HELP* your horse, please be skeptical. You'll likely not be doing your horse any favors and might actually set him up for orthopedic stresses that will cause greater problems down the line. The best thing for any athlete is working slowly to build their muscles, abilities and talent. Can anyone really expect a horse to be helped through mechanical training and shoeing techniques? Those methods do not help him change but simply masks the problem by encumbering his natural movement.

Many people simply avoid the show ring as a response to the problem of mechanical and abusive training. But I not only enjoy showing but see significant value and potential benefit to sound shows where quality judging rewards the naturally brilliant and correct gaits. How better to improve a breed than to set up competition for those very characteristics that will indeed improve both the athletic abilities and conformation of a versatile utility and pleasure horse? So what is the solution? The only way is to change the game by insisting on standards of judging and purity of gait that cannot be produced or enhanced mechanically. To train judges to recognize and reward gaiting standards that does *not depend* on an artificially *forced, framed or fixed* way of going. Even to penalize those horses moving in a mechanical or laboring way that indicates unscrupulous training practices.

The time has come for true horsemanship to return to the Walking Horse world! It is time for our wonderful breed to be celebrated for its brilliant and natural abilities and versatility. I am not a person who condemns showing in general for all of the ills because not all show organizations defend the status quo. There are those Horse Industry Organizations that protect everything bad in their own misguided attempt to promote the breed. However there are others adamant in their promotion of the natural horse and my friends there is nothing I'd rather do than watch brilliantly correct horses working in comfort and unity with their riders. It makes my heart sing and makes me proud to support these organizations.

How can you and I make a difference? Well the ugly truth is the only voice each of us has is the way we spend our money and in what breed organizations we support with our dollars. Period! You can talk to people 'till you turn blue in the face, but it's where your money goes that gives your feelings a voice. I know many people claim that performance shows are the only thing close to them to show in. There are several options for you if you're in that situation. It may not be easier (probably won't be) but you will have control of your voice again.

1. You can organize a small group to put on your own fun show and affiliate with a sound organization that promotes the values and training you support.

2. You can request and sponsor gaited horse classes within local all-breed shows and provide them with rules of sound horse

organizations that you wish their judges to judge your classes by.

3. You save your nickels and travel hours across state(s) to patronize those shows that do sponsor and support those organizations you feel adhere to your training and showing values.

If you wish to show your pleasure Walking Horse, then CHOOSE YOUR SHOWS carefully. Do your homework. Today we are blessed with show circuits and judging programs that not only recognize true and correct gait, but will penalize those horses who appear to have been trained through mechanical means. This is the best thing to happen to gaited horses in many years and I highly recommend both Friends of Sound Horses, Inc. as well as the National Walking Horse Association for embracing and protecting the naturally gaited Walking Horses. There are often local organizations and clubs that sponsor shows which actively prevent mechanical horses from being rewarded and promoted. All such organizations are helping people to seek alternative and sound gait solutions and finally giving not just Walking Horses, but all the gaited breeds a place to show their sound, naturally trained horses. It may mean driving a few more hours and even an overnight rather than the convenience of a local show every weekend.

If you have a local show circuit or charitable groups that put on gaited shows every year but they are affiliating with an HIO that does not support the USDA and enforce the Horse Protection Act, or it does not promote fair judging standards that promote real training solutions over fixes, then you need to keep looking, or lobby their show management to affiliate with these sound HIO's. Appeal to their need to cover costs by offering to find sponsorships and bringing in other pleasure horse enthusiasts if they are willing to consider this alternative affiliation.

SUITABILITY FOR THE SHOW RING

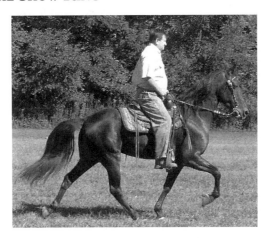

Gary Lane - WindsweptStables.net

If you are serious about wanting to show you should consider choosing a horse with the potential to develop. I believe ANY Walking Horse can find a place to show successfully, as mentioned earlier, because if you can get your horse CORRECT in his gaits you're halfway there, but if you wish to compete at the top levels of both regional and national competitions your horse should have the natural talent to develop. You should not try to make a horse into something his breeding and conformation does not support. That is the road to frustration for you both and may very well cause you to be unhappy with a wonderful pleasure horse that simply should remain just that, a pleasure horse. There is nothing wrong with polishing the gaits of any horse as long as you are enjoying the journey and do not define your success by the ribbons you bring home. I say "go for it".

I've always advised people that there are two essentials abilities a top show horse should be bred with: big stride and natural looseness. Most everything else can be trained and polished through patient saddle time. But even those horses that lack these talents can often find success in the challenge of versatility events.

STRIDE

I find I can best evaluate stride potential from both conformation and by watching a horse move at a slow walk on a lead ***without a rider.*** So often a rider unintentionally hampers a horse's natural stride potential. I want to evaluate a horse while he's moving at a relaxed loose trail walk where he demonstrates a sweeping backend showing about 12-14 inches of overstride with each step at low energy with even timing. This is quite respectable stride and tells me he can be taught to extend to even greater reach. I also review the depth and angle of the gaskin which will give an indication of his natural ability to reach beneath as well as behind.

Your horse needs to have the basic conformation to stride long and deep to be competitive at top levels of the pleasure divisions. If the barebones talent is there it can be developed to extend and strengthen. Most horses can be taught to maximize whatever natural striding ability they have, and you should probably plan on adding several inches to their relaxed leadline stride with some patient instruction. You should not, however, expect to take a horse with 4 inches of isochronal overstride on the lead and expand that to 30 inches of overstride under saddle. That's neither reasonable nor fair to expect of

LOOSENESS

Looseness is a difficult characteristic to describe and quantify, but once you learn to see it you'll always be able to see it. It's a fluid flow of energy in a neutral and relaxed way where the horse is balancing equally on all four corners. It's seen in horses that almost seem to crawl across the ground rolling their shoulders, nodding their head and almost lumbering with their back ends. I sometimes say they move in an almost catlike crawling motion, while using their headnod. Old timers would say they appear to "almost fall apart as they walk." I say they appear kind of lazy, like they don't waste energy without a reason,

your horse. See **Extending and Developing Stride** later in this chapter.

rolling from hoof to hoof with natural non-suspended carriage.

However you wish to describe it these are horses that have the potential to learn to extend both energy levels and speed *WHILE MAINTAINING THAT LOOSENESS*. That natural inclination to maintain their looseness while increasing energy and stride produces the brilliance of a natural show gait. When developed with care to avoid the essential tension resulting from force will help preserve that looseness, while any application of the three F's of force, frame or fix will likely degrade the very looseness we're seeking.

OTHER BENEFICIAL CONFORMATION FEATURES

A solidly built topline from poll to tail dock is essential to any horse needing to maintain a neutral carriage with a rider on board. I spoke at length about needed saddle fit and back comfort, but if a horse has a neck or back conformation weakness such as extreme sway or roaching he will almost always need to brace his dorsal muscles to compensate and support that weakness. The result of this need to brace dorsal muscles invariably pushes these horses to pace, or at best to rack. Sometimes careful shim padding can help relieve topline stresses tremendously, but attention will need to be taken to address this to help your horse achieve a fluidly rolling walk with any speed.

Good width of shoulder not only indicates the horse has the ability to carry a significant load, it also tells us he should be able to release and reach with them. Just as you will rarely find a baseball player with narrow shoulders,

a horse that needs to stride out should have significant width to assist this desired movement. FYI: many in the performance horse industry believe a more narrow shoulder allows the horse to lift and flog a stacked hoof high. I do not advocate breeding a narrow shoulder for this type of animation and feel it is a disservice to these horses to promote this conformation. Not only does this detract from his forward reaching ability, but a narrow shoulder tends to lend itself to hoof problems in a horse that by necessity maintains a base wide stance. They will load to the inside hoof wall creating an imbalance in hoof growth patterns that require constant maintenance to manage.

Beyond these attributes, sound conformation for any saddle horse includes traditional characteristics of short back, straight legs and depth of chest.

Developing Natural Stride for a Show Gait

For a naturally brilliant walking horse stride must be maximized and developed, for it is at this deep-working extended stride that a horse utilizes his greatest backend engagement, counterbalances with a deep and prominent headnod as well as a lightly floating front end. All of these add polish and shine to a horse's more common gait. Natural stride extension is something each horse can be taught, *but it is not an overnight occurrence and you should plan on enjoying the journey.* If you focus only on the end goal you will tend to become frustrated those days your horse is just not making as much progress as you hoped for. Your frustration may very well interfere with your companionable working relationship with your horse. This is a long-term project, not a quick alteration. The good news is that every year you ride a horse in correct form he becomes stronger and surer in his gait and gets more brilliant as well.

Many sound trainers will advocate intentionally pushing the flat shod Walking Horse into a pace to break loose the backend. Basically this is how they have learned to maximize stride. *I'm not a big fan of ever intentionally pushing a horse toward off-gait.* I'd much rather he develops his brilliance at the isochronal walking posture and strengthen the default gait rather than force a lateral timing and the hollow posture that usually goes with it. Not to mention all the inherent problems in deliberately asking for a gait that introduces tension into the topline. In any case, I am totally convinced that if you understand how, you can actually get *more* extension at the flatfoot walk than at the pace. It does take a light and practiced seat to encourage this starting with your horse rating his speed to your seat.

What I want is for people to use this same seat of your pants riding to encourage your horse to extend and really reach with his walking stride. You do this by thinking bigger, not faster. We want to encourage our horses with everything inside us to be big and bold in their walks, to be deep, regular and even with their headnod (remember the headnod drives the backend) and swing that stride slow and deep. I won't fool you, it will take practice, but I promise that if you're persistent *your horse will start reaching within himself to follow your lead in this dance.*

I also recommend a careful use of the one rein half-halt along with a driving seat. Some would call it a connecting half-halt, or a very light leg yield with hindquarter redirection. Much like the shoulder-in helps force a horse to release and roll out of his shoulder, the haunches out movement will help a horse to release the backend stride into a single deep step. I have found that when I apply a light one-rein capture or half-halt paired with a light driving leg in the back position on the same side, the horse tends to take a slightly lateral step out with the opposite hind leg, giving you one stride that is deeper and longer than he previously was using in his straight track. If you can then release the one-rein capture at the precise instant you feel this longer stride behind, totally freeing his head and keep with the driving leg to encourage his forward motion with your seat he can learn to carry this longer reach for several strides. You do this again and again during your training session and the horse begins to understand you're asking for that deeper stride. Once you learn how to use this, you have a valuable tool in asking your horse to reach deep within himself for maximum stride while he maintains his released and neutral walking topline. You're not pushing him into a pace that increases his topline tension to try to get stride. You're teaching him correct form at the same time you're asking him to reach within himself and extend his stride.

By Anita J Howe

FEEL THE GAIT

The bottom line for show training: you cannot correct or train what you do not understand or cannot feel. If you cannot feel the posture, balance, attitude and movement of the horse you will have great difficulty in trying to encourage your horse when he's moving correctly as well as correct your horse when he's not. So in the interest of further helping you understand how correct movement feels from the saddle (most of us do not have mirrors allowing us to watch as we ride) I want to discuss how the deep, showy walking gaits should feel to the rider.

First understand that the front and back supporting pair of legs should be off sequence to each other at the isochronal four beat walk. Meaning when the back hooves are mid-stride the front will be at their weight transfer moment. Conversely when the front is mid-stride the back end should be at its weight transfer moment. What this means from the saddle is that as the backend is pushing as the front is lifting. When the front end is stretching with both hooves on the ground, the backend pushes ease slightly.

Another key feature to feel is the headnod counterbalancing with the backend. As the backend is at its weight transfer moment with both hooves on the ground the headnod should be at its lowest point just as the base of the neck and shoulders are *LIFTED* to their highest point. This lightness and lift at the shoulders is essential to a quality walking gait. The horse should keep his backend engaged and pushing with solid sweeping and alternating long strides. If ever he feels like his shoulders are dropping down or sinking he will tend to bring his head up when his shoulders sink. At this point your horse is only a heartbeat away from disengaging into a jigging backend.

What all of these alternating movements feel like is a front-to-back rocking motion under the saddle with the head dropping as the shoulders lift and the head lifting and the shoulders drop. It is also important to note that as long as the backend is engaged and sweeping it should feel quiet with no lifted jogging or jigging. Also the front-to-back rolling motion is a good thing for those who wish to exhibit their Walking Horses because the deeper the walk the stronger and deeper that front-to-back roll will be at the slower flatfoot walk. So you should encourage this motion by releasing your lumbar area and moving with your horse. The roll or rock should always remain soft and easy to sit. If the ride ever begins to feel jerky then it indicates the horse is starting to sink heavy on his fore and either his shoulders are jamming his front hooves into the ground or he's getting diagonal in his timing and moving more toward a foxtrot. Both of these off gaits feel jerky to the rider. If the head is coming up most likely he's getting hollow, pacey and heavy. If the head is level and the nose is reaching out he's most likely sliding a little into the zone of the foxtrot. Either way, jerky is not a good thing to feel in the saddle for a quality walking gait.

I tell people the movement through the topline of a well engaged Walking Horse should feel like a wave moving from back to front on the horse and they need to get in sync with that movement; to ride the wave. I've heard other riders describe it as an inchworm kind of feel.

So let's do a recap of what you should feel:

- Quiet and strong pushing backend
- Front to back rolling movement
- Light and floating on the front coupled with a looseness through the shoulder
- Lift and drop at the shoulders in alternating movement to the headnod
- Isochronal timing of hoof beats

To help your horse you will need to

encourage him to drop his head down as deep as he can with each reach of backend stride. We want him to stride deep underneath himself and the best way promote this deep stride is to allow him to drop his headnod deeply in counterbalance. As he drops his head his ventral muscles are contracting and pulling his back leg under in a singular motion. If your hands are unintentionally interfering with the head dropping down by too much contact on the reins you are, in reality, inhibiting his ability to reach well under. So stay out of his mouth and encourage him to nod his head deeply.

A Commitment to Show

If you've decided your horse has the talent and you truly wish to develop his abilities for the sound show ring, you will need to make a personal commitment to develop him at his default walking gait for many months. He needs to work at extending his stride and increasing his walking energy while maintaining a neutral core in loose release. This takes patience and persistence and you must be willing to give him the time to develop. Otherwise you'll find yourself looking for those very same quick fixes so popular among performance industry trainers. Somewhere around the 4-6 months point of training a very naturally loose and big strided Walking Horse can be set on a path to develop his show potential. I normally have a very honest conversation with owners who may be interested and give them my professional opinion whether this horse A) has the ability, B) has the correct temperament and C) whether the owner has the desire and commitment to proceed. Until all three of these are present you should not consider your horse a show horse.

There is nothing wrong with admitting that your horse is not suitable for the show ring or that you do not wish to show. I also believe that most owners would rather hear an honest evaluation up front before investing the time, effort and money into such a project. Conversely if you have a very talented horse, I believe there's nothing finer that allowing him the opportunity to develop his shine. Whether it's your personal time or that of a paid trainer, training is an investment in your horse and as such should increase his value for the rest of his days.

While there are no real deadlines for making this decision, if you allow him to progress to his faster gaits without extensive foundation work at his default walking gait then you could possibly create some bad habits that would entail additional time to overcome later.

Straightness and Balance

Balance and straightness are essentials for any horse of any breed. Balance to me means a horse traveling with fluid impulsion from back to front and never being ridden out of his mouth or in any way from front to back. The rider must respect that the horse needs to give us his brilliance voluntarily to not only preserve the looseness described above but to preserve his balance and backend impulsion and enable him to bloom on the front from a strong push and engagement behind.

Always begin your training at the trail walk, described as default walk, and whenever your horse begins to lose the gait in anyway, bring him back to his default walk. Eventually as he becomes more stable and set in his timing and balance you can transition up to the flatfoot walk as his new default walk, but that is only as the horse is developing and should not be expected of the beginner horse.

Straightness is as essential as balance. Straightness to me means a symmetrical gait where the horse travels evenly with both sides of his body. If your horse, for any reason, uses one side consistently stronger than the other his gait is far from the only thing to suffer. If he exhibits more stiffness and less suppleness on one side, he must become more even and straight both for his gait as well as his future orthopedic soundness. Just as you and I need to be aware of our straightness for orthopedic health, so does your horse. The quadrupeds have an even more complex system of gait than the bipeds, and when lameness or favoring in one quadrant occurs the remaining quadrants must and will invariably compensate. Often that very compensation will cause an even greater soreness and discomfort than the original injury or pain. For instance an uneven saddle tree pushing into one shoulder of the horse can cause both the opposite fore as well as the laterally paired hind to compensate and try to avoid rolling and reaching as far out of that shoulder. The other legs fill in and allow the horse to reduce the range of motion and weight bearing of the uncomfortable shoulder in a protective movement. Suddenly you now have uneven use of the forelegs, but also uneven use of the hind legs and have potential for orthopedic problems in the shoulders, the lower neck, as well as the LS joint of the spine.

All of this was a result of one bad place on a saddle tree.

I have personal experience with knee injuries and found I became aware of it because I had learned to compensate through the other leg and the lower back and was experiencing discomfort in those areas. All of these connected areas begin to be over-taxed because the skeletal structure is designed to support our weight and balance with minimal effort *WHEN IT IS STRAIGHT AND EVEN SIDE TO SIDE*. Anytime we are slumped, or leaning we overburden one area to compensate for another. Our horse is the same way. They are designed to carry themselves in a variety of postures and balances as long as they are straight side to side allowing each quadrant to carry its share of the burden equally. Our job is to interfere with that balance and straightness *AS LITTLE AS POSSIBLE*. To fit the saddle and sit the horse straight, with level shoulders and our own weight being as little distraction to our horse as possible. Have you ever ridden a bicycle with a passenger sitting behind? If so you can understand how essential it is for that passenger to remain balanced and to move with you and the bicycle. This is just how we must learn to balance with our horse and not distort or throw off his straightness.

DIVISIONS FOR THE PLEASURE WALKING HORSE

I am going to briefly delve into a realm that most people normally leave up to the show circuit to define. My reasons for doing so are to attempt to influence those circuits who promote a natural horse toward bringing consistency to their judging systems. So please do not take this as specific guide for any particular show or circuit, but more about my feelings regarding these often obscure division definitions set up by the ruling organizations. I've come to the conclusion that we have some serious confusion occurring between exhibitors and those who develop, refine and judge the rules about these divisions.

I want to stress that we need to pay more attention the *reasons* for having divisions. It's not about simply giving more horses more places to show. It's *NOT* about setting up more options for competition at a championship show. What it should be about is celebrating the great diversity and versatility of our breed. There are Walking Horses that can sprint, that can jump, that can herd cows or negotiate obstacles. There are likewise Walking Horses that can strut with elegance and brilliance or can move out with a balanced trail demeanor, or faultlessly execute a dressage pattern. The PURPOSE of the divisions is to give each of these types a level playing field of competition, while defining different judging parameters for each based on way of going rather than how much mechanical influence is being applied.

A Trail Pleasure horse should never be considered LESS HORSE than an English Pleasure horse. It has different qualities with different demeanor and carriage. A Country Pleasure horse is likewise NOT less of a horse, it is a horse to be admired and encouraged because of his willingness, calmness, smooth gait and great mind. We should focus on what these horses do that we want to celebrate and develop divisional parameters along those lines. When we do this we can begin to develop consistency between show and judging programs that will not be so confusing to spectators as well as exhibitors. This will not only provide more consistency, but help discourage judges from taking the easy choice of biggest is best, while disregarding how correct the gait is. It will further encourage exhibitors to pay more attention to their horse's way of going rather than how he is shod.

So far, only two organizations have been bold enough to mandate that walking gaits are to be correct, first and foremost. That a horse with less animation may still win over a horse with bigger stride and animation, if their gait is more authentic and correct. We must reward correctness above animation if we wish to preserve its unique and foundation qualities. These organizations are Friends of Sound Horses, Inc. and the National Walking Horse Association, and I highly recommend support for both if you wish to show a natural Walking Horse. There are many hard working individuals within both of these organizations that dedicate a tremendous amount of personal time, effort and funds to promote the correct and brilliant Tennessee Walking Horse.

Please note that my opinion for divisions **has nothing to do with what shoes are on the horse.** The purpose of the horse does not change with the shoes he's got on. We must distance ourselves from the entire notion of shoeing for gait enhancement. It is the road to nowhere for this breed. I personally do *NOT* believe in shoeing with anything other than a 10-11 oz. keg shoe, and even then only if the horse needs that support, and you won't need to either if you support shows that affiliate through the judging programs I've mentioned above. I have won multiple national championship and grand-championship titles on horses wearing keg shoes as well as barefoot horses.

The primary divisions for clarification are:

- Pleasure or Lite-shod divisions
- Trail Pleasure divisions
- Country Pleasure divisions

PLEASURE OR LITE-SHOD DIVISIONS are for those horses who are the epitome of the natural show horse. They are the *BRILLIANTLY BOLD AND BEAUTIFUL* horses who strut with brio and look at me attitude. These horses should have the deepest stride, headnod and biggest front end float. They should always remain true in form by reaching well out of their shoulders and never jog or thump their chest with too much knee action that sacrifices their forward reach. An evenly timed overstride greater than 18 inches should be typical and reflect a deep stride in the range of 8 to 10 feet from point of pickup to plant relative to the overall size of the horse.

These horses should show us a truly productive headnod that works to drive their deep backend in a pumping counterbalanced motion originating from the shoulders while the attitude and angle of the poll does not change. The headnod should correctly dip to its lowest point as each rear hoof plants. This correct movement should NEVER be sacrificed for speed that degrades its form. The running walk should reflect a distinctive increase of both speed and tempo as the horse extends their correct flatfoot walking form, and timing should *never* deviate from even and isochronal timing.

A Trail Pleasure horse is just that... a pleasure for the trail rider. He will not usually have as long of a stride and probably not as deep of a headnod as those horses in the Pleasure division. What he will have is a more balanced front-to-back carriage and four cornered gait that eats up the trail while allowing a more natural and level head carriage for better viewing of potential obstacles ahead. He should demonstrate the ability and willingness to drop into a slow, relaxed trail walk at the brief cue of his rider; moving forward in this waiting for further instructions mode without being actively held back. He should back willingly and respond lightly to leg cues of his rider working in partnership. I wish to point out that the Pleasure division horse is still suitable for trail riding, but the Trail Pleasure division is for those horses that carry themselves in a manner that says "I have a purpose beyond the show ring!" While some people may not agree with me, I personally prefer a slightly shorter strided horse on the more rugged trails that tend to keep speeds down to the flatfoot walk and the trail walk. At these slower speeds those horses with the huge stride will tend to have big front-to-back rolling motion from the saddle that will not be as comfortable for the rider. Also those huge striding steps are often not as sure footed as the more stable 6 to 7 foot stride and 10 – 12inch *EVENLY TIMED* overstride.

You can easily teach a longer strided horse to shorten his stride and become more sure footed if you wish to ride them on the trail by practicing through Cavaletti that are more set close together. But many people who own horses suitable for the Pleasure divisions are reluctant to ask them to shorten their stride for any reason if they enjoy showing.

The Country Pleasure horses are the one division where perfection of timing and form are not as prized. The characteristics most desirable in a country pleasure horse are willingness, calmness, and smoothness of gait, easy transitions and responsiveness. As long as the gait is smooth and four beat it is less concerning whether or not it is text-book and precisely correct. Huge stride is likewise less of a priority, and may even be somewhat detrimental to the smooth ride if the horse extends beyond a certain level of comfort for the rider. Remember we are looking for a horse with different priorities; a horse that travels in a willing and comfortable gait. A horse that is sure footed and moves in balanced self carriage that requires very little rider support to stay smooth in his gait. The epitome of the Country Pleasure horse is versatile, making transitions of both speed and direction smoothly, and with little support. He backs readily with little pulling and no force with a lowered head and showing obvious diagonal pairing during the reinback that indicates a properly rounded topline.

What I want everyone to think about long before they take their horse to a show is what type of horse do I think my horse is? Where do I see him or her being most successful and what division does he/she best represent? Then spend the weeks in advance of the show preparing and polishing the characteristics most desired for that division. Practice just as though you are in the show ring, all the way through the lineup and reinback. Get your horse used to the routine and find out if he has any unexpected issues with standing relaxed on a loose rein in the lineup, if he can negotiate a neck rein turn for western classes or even a rein back with a 360 haunch turn as some show circuits like for their western disciplines. I do not get caught up at all about parking out... and actually much prefer this particular tradition be abandoned. I love to see horses standing square and solid, waiting patiently and relaxed until asked for something else, no matter the discipline or division.

Chapter 16 - Rehabilitating the Performance Horse

Unfortunately there are a large percentage of the pleasure walking horses being purchased every season that have originated from culls of the performance show world breeding and training barns. Many of these horses will be quite natural in their gaits which, believe it or not, could be one possible reason they are being culled. Some have washed out of the puppy-mill big lick or performance training programs, while some may have developed lameness issues from being pushed too hard as young yearlings. Still others have simply been mentally stressed to the point where they are no longer willing to be ridden or harbor a perpetual fear of humans. Whatever the reason, many horses that come out of that industry have issues to be dealt with. Most are what I classify as special needs horses.

Many will claim that the culls are the lucky ones, and I guess it varies with each horse and how well it has coped with the training methods it has been exposed to so far. Just like children that have been subjected to harsh or institutional environments, these horses are in need of a great deal of love and patience from whoever purchases them. What they do have in their favor is their natural calmness and inherent desire to get along that has been fostered within this breed for many generations. Very few Walking Horses (and I've been exposed to hundreds within this breed) have demonstrated any ability to become aggressive even when harshly mistreated. It is simply not part of their psyche. I've always referred to Walking Horses as the golden retrievers of the horse world, and they will tolerate so much mistreatment and neglect while never exhibiting what I would consider a healthy self-preservation defense mechanism. When pushed to the limits of their tolerance, some of them simply withdraw or become frightened and shy creatures around all humans.

I will say that if you have the love and patience within you to invest yourself into these beautiful animals, you have a special place in Heaven, in my opinion. But just as an abrupt and harsh teacher will have difficulty reaching a special-needs child, an owner or trainer who is not patient and in tune to a horse's emotional state will have difficulty reaching and successfully working to rehabilitate an emotionally scarred horse.

We have a huge advantage working in our favor with these horses in that even through any harsh treatment *they still want to get along and please*. What we need to be aware of is their worry and hesitant ability to trust us. They want to trust us, but their experiences have taught them not to. So we must earn their trust by showing them *we have their comfort and best interest at heart at all times*. Your biggest tool will be your patience and persistence. Your calm understanding that your new horse will have good days and bad days will help you to not get frustrated or discouraged. Remember they read our body language and frustration may be mistaken as anger toward them.

One of the biggest problems that people encounter with ex-performance horses is their thought that we always want them to move out and move fast. This is a result from being performance shod and pushed to work hard up and down the training barn aisles. Straight line forward movement is almost always their only training and the majority of that is down a barn aisle, turn around to the left and back up the barn aisle. I've seen horses that have been ridden under saddle for a year or more that have never learned how to turn right! They are naturally resistant to move when first shod with stacks and action devices and rather than being taught to respond to any leg cues a riding crop is often applied liberally when they show any reluctance. Is it any wonder that they quickly figure out the sooner they move out when someone climbs into the saddle the less they'll feel the crop or spurs? Add to that a horse's natural inclination to run away from whatever scares them and you have a recipe for a very forward, almost out of control horse. To further complicate matters, while being gigged to move out they are often yanked hard in the mouth onto a severe bit. So be understanding and be patient. I will not go into any horror stories here. This is not venue, nor is that the focus of this book.

When you get one of these forward horses I recommend you begin working with them in a small arena or paddock. *Do your bit training at a standstill with a mild bit* so that your horse learns that first a bit might actually be kind rather than abusive. The second thing they need to realize is that any kind of connection does NOT mean take off and move as hard as you can. Teach them to lower their head and slowly walk out. If they still want to be squirty and forward you will need to introduce them to a one rein stop and

keep turning them into the rail until they slow down to a trail walk. It is very important to use a mild bit and to ***always release any contact after they slow or when you've finished turning***. These horses must begin to realize that a slow walk is the desired default and that a bit is not always punishing. Build their trust by constantly reassuring them. I like to use treats liberally with these horses after teaching them that teeth are not allowed.

Tip: Let me briefly say that I am a firm believer in treating horses as a little extra reward and incentive. It is a method of quickly letting them know when they do something especially well. Many trainers will discourage you from treating out of your hand because of the risk of a bite, but my philosophy is if you don't want your horse to bite, train him that it is unacceptable! I offer the treat on the palm of my hand and if I feel any teeth at all I grab his soft nose, digging in my fingernails quickly, briefly and hard so it's as though my hand is biting him back on that most sensitive area. I immediately offer my bare palm again and again. I allow lips and tongue, but never any teeth. Within a few minutes you can teach a horse that biting is not and will not be tolerated. After that it becomes a non-issue. This is not a new concept for any horse since his mother had to teach him it was not acceptable to bite when his first little teeth came in at a few days old. He can easily learn this lesson without getting his feelings hurt. You will not want to overuse treats because of the risk of a horse becoming pushy. Once I have established that they get a treat as a reward then I only offer them when the horse has accomplished something significant, or had his light bulb moment of epiphany.

With the forward horse we want to use the positive reward and reinforcement as much as possible. By learning to relax, release his topline and slow down to a trail walk as his default speed he will become not only a calmer and less squirty horse, but a better thinker and less spooky as well. All of these are beneficial for a compatible partnership and training. Remember that the performance horse has been taught to be a forward horse so cut him a lot of slack since he's only doing what he thinks you want.

Most, if not all performance horses have also been TAUGHT to pace. Yes, that's right, taught to pace. So be prepared to deal with that also. In the majority of cases they are not any pacier due to their conformation than many other pleasure horses, but indeed most know how to pace quite well for the reasons above as well as the ones mentioned in the chapter on **Curing the Pace**. There is the firm belief by most performance horse trainers that the only way to get extended stride out of a horse is to pace him out, and anytime they seem to be squaring up too soon, they'll pace them a little more in an attempt to keep their stride at maximum reach. Well you can imagine that I'm not in agreement that method. Remember the **Illusion of Overstride** lesson? I don't know if these trainers really believe this or if they're just trying to get everyone else to buy into what they're selling. It makes no sense to me to teach a horse to be off gaited because

you want him to extend his reach. If you want him to reach and extend then train him to reach and extend. Let him develop the strong muscles needed to carry that extension while he's actually working a correct gait.

Another belief for teaching them to pace is that the horse must have very lateral timing to carry the weight of the action devices used without squaring up too much. A naturally timed horse would be pushed into a trot if you applied all the weight of the mechanical shoeing used for performance horses, which is why I mentioned that the very naturally gaited horses are frequently the first ones to be culled and you can often find very talented horses being sold off.

So if you purchase an ex-performance horse be prepared to deal with his worry, his forwardness, his lack of trust and his pacing. And always remember that underneath all these rough spots, **which are man-made** just like his incorrect gait, there still resides a wonderful, loving animal that will give his heart and soul to please you and to be the recipient of your love. He deserves better and I sure hope each and every one of them gets that opportunity to shine.